S0-AGC-424

The Myth of Safe Sex

The Tragic Consequences
of Violating God's Plan

The Myth of Safe Sex

The Tragic Consequences
of Violating God's Plan

by

Dr. John Ankerberg

and

Dr. John Weldon

Moody Press

Chicago

© 1993 by
John F. Ankerberg & John F. Weldon

All rights reserved. No part of this publication may be reproduced,
stored in a retrieval system, or transmitted in any form by any means,
electronic, mechanical, photocopy, recording, or otherwise, without
the prior written permission of the publishers, except for brief quotations in critical reviews or articles.

All Scripture quotations, unless indicated, are taken from the *Holy
Bible: New International Version*, copyright 1973, 1978, 1984 by Inter-
national Bible Society. Used by permission of Zondervan Publishing
House. All rights reserved.

Scripture quotations marked (NASB) are taken from the *American
Standard Bible*, copyright 1960, 1962, 1963, 1968, 1971, 1972, 1973,
1975, and 1977 by The Lockman Foundation and are used by permission.

The Ankerberg Theological Research Institute
Chattanooga, Tennessee 37411

ISBN 0–8024–5639–1

1 3 5 7 9 10 8 6 4 2

Printed in the United States of America

Contents

Note to the Reader

The delicate and often controversial subject matter of this book is such that it will touch every reader's life in one way or another. It may also tend to cause a strong emotional reaction, either positively or negatively.

The authors' reaction can be seen in what might be considered as "editorial" statements in some chapters. These are not necessarily indictments of individuals who may not agree with us. Nor should they be used as an excuse to ignore the message of this book. We have well-grounded feelings about this subject and have not hesitated to state them clearly.

The facts are clear. Something must be done soon to reverse society's moral decline and stop the spread of AIDS, and it is obvious that current government and health service programs are not doing the job. Thus, we have attempted to critically examine the sexual mores of our culture in the hopes that our readers will see anew the extent of the problem and attempt to bring change where needed in their own communities. In a subject so broad, we have undoubtedly stepped on some toes. We ask the reader's indulgence and understanding in our attempt to deal forthrightly with a difficulty subject.

Our criticism is not to be construed as meaning that we have no compassion or concern for those who are suffering the consequences of their actions. As sinners ourselves, we have great empathy for the fact that sin "so easily entangles us" (Hebrews 12:1 NASB) and believe wholeheartedly that "judgment without mercy will be shown to anyone who has not been merciful. Mercy triumphs over judgment!" (James 2:13).

However, there comes a time when the welfare of society as a whole is at such risk that certain things must be said that not all will understand. We hope it will be evident that not only are we concerned with the welfare of individuals; we are also concerned with the welfare of the nation.

Introduction

The ocean swell from an earthquake in Chile or Japan will travel thousands of miles before hitting Hawaii or California hours later. A tidal wave, or *tsunami,* is a truly phenomenal event. Often beginning far underneath the ocean through volcanic activity, the upsurge of land mass displaces water, which begins traveling in all directions. Once a tidal wave begins, no force on earth can stop it.

As it travels along the ocean's surface, it is undetectable as it silently passes under ships. At this point, the wave is only a few inches high. But the tidal surge is there and traveling at speeds of up to five hundred miles per hour.

Today, a different *tsunami* is rippling undetected offshore. The often unconsidered, but rapidly traveling, consequences of the sexual revolution are the social tidal waves of the twenty-first century. Some tomorrow they will crash on shore. Exactly when and where, and with what consequence, no one can say.

Nothing is free, least of all sex, which is bound to our deepest sources of energy, identity, and emotion. Sex can be cheapened, of course, but then, inevitably, it becomes extremely costly to the society as a whole. . . . When sex is devalued, propagandized, and deformed, as at present, the quality of our lives declines and our social fabric deteriorates.

George Gilder, *Sexual Suicide*

The sexual revolution has ripped apart the social fabric of American society. As a result, sexual confusion has spread disease throughout the culture, destroying families (the number of marriages which end in divorce has skyrocketed from 6% to 51% since the beginning of this century), promoting violent sexual crimes against women and children (rape has increased over 526% since the 1960s and child abuse has become a national shame) and fostering an epidemic growth of sexual diseases such as herpes, gonorrhea, chlamydia, PID, bacterial vaginosis, trichomoniasis, hepatitis B, hepatitis C, syphilis, and AIDS. Our media, schools and government have become propagandists, promoters and protectors of sexual deviance. The old Judeo-Christian taboos have been cast aside, and our young men and women have been set adrift in a sea of uncertainty.

Movie Critic Ted Baehr, *Movieguide*

1

What Everyone Should Know About the Cause and Cure of Sexual Promiscuity

The Legacy of the Sexual Revolution

Most of America is familiar with Lauren Chapin, the actress who played Cathy Anderson in the popular television series "Father Knows Best." But according to several sources, such as the *Phoenix Gazette*, as Cathy grew up in the real world, she encountered a life far different from that portrayed in the TV show. Searching for happiness, she recalls, "I slept with many, many people trying to find love, to find self-worth. And the more people I slept with the less self-worth I had." As the years passed, before she became a Christian, Lauren Chapin suffered the results of searching for love and meaning through casual sex. Her involvement with numerous lovers, drugs, and Hollywood's "fast lane" (which she termed a "death zone") proved costly. It affected her health, brought eight miscarriages, and resulted in time spent in a mental hospital, and even prison.[1]

Many people are like Lauren. They believe that having sex will bring them the affection, love, and purpose in life they now lack. But instead of happiness and contentment, it often results in decreased self-esteem, pain, rejection, and sometimes tragedy.

Some people today don't think we have a social problem in the area of the nation's sexual behavior. They continue to call for sexual liberty to counteract "repressive" and "puritanical" attitudes. But we do have a problem, and it is one of the most serious we face.

THE SEXUAL EXPLOSION

Many regional and national studies have revealed similar findings. For good or ill, the generation of the "sexual revolution" has transferred its sexual values to the larger society and even to its own children. Billions of dollars have been spent on sex education and family planning programs that have resulted only in a dramatic increase in promiscuous sexual activity and its consequences. *The Washington Post* revealed "that half of U.S. girls have now had intercourse by the age of fifteen."[2]

A major research study of eleven million teenage boys showed that 66 percent had had sex, the average age of the first encounter was sixteen, and by eighteen the average boy had had sex with five different girls.[3]

A New York polling firm supplied forty-one questions, describing the "average" adolescent, to 1,300 students in sixteen high schools, 1600 students in ten colleges, and 500 parents of teens in twelve cities. This and other studies found that:

- 57 percent lost their virginity in high school.
- 79 percent lost their virginity by the end of college.
- 33 percent of high school students had sex one to four times a month.[4]
- 53 percent of fifteen to nineteen year olds had been involved sexually; 58 percent of teen girls had two or more sex partners.[5]

Senate Bill 2394 of the state of California discussed some of the statistics of teenage sexual behavior in that state:

- Sixty-five percent of male teens and 44 percent of females have had sexual intercourse by eighteen.
- Every year one in seven teens contracts a sexually transmitted disease (STD).
- The teenage pregnancy rate for California's fifteen to nineteen year olds increased by almost 33 percent from 1970 to 1985.
- The abortion rate for teens fifteen to nineteen has more than tripled in the same period.[6]

By age nineteen, 75 percent of unmarried women have had or are having sexual intercourse.[7]

Unfortunately, statistics on sexual activity (or anything else) can be difficult to assess.[8] They are easily manipulated and can be misleading, so we encourage caution in accepting the above figures as absolutes.

A Louis Harris poll showed that 90 percent of teens admitted they had become promiscuous simply because of *perceived* peer pressure. Of those who had sex, 80 percent said they felt they had been drawn into sex too soon. Regret often causes such teens to cut back on sexual behavior; unfortunately, teens who have had sex only once are classified as "sexually active," inflating the teenage promiscuity rate. . . . Regarding the relative inactivity and return to abstinence among teens who had had sexual intercourse, it is realistic to promote "secondary virginity." As Dr. James Ford notes, "These figures indicate that secondary virginity is not all that rare among teenagers. In other words, an appreciable percentage of unmarried teenagers who have experienced premarital intercourse are not currently 'sexually active.'"[9]

But the teens who are sexually active still number in the millions—and even if some figures are inflated, no one can deny that a serious problem exists.

Former Secretary of Education William J. Bennett, in a speech to the National School Board Association, revealed some sobering facts:

- More than one million teenage girls become pregnant each year, and 40 percent of today's fourteen-year-old girls will become pregnant by the time they are nineteen.
- Teenage pregnancy rates are at or near an all-time high. The 25 percent decline in birth rates between 1970 and 1984 was due to a doubling of the abortion rate during that period. More than 400,000 teenage girls have abortions each year.

Bennett himself confessed, "These numbers are an irrefutable indictment of sex education's effectiveness in reducing teenage sexual activity and pregnancies."[10]

According to a national survey listing items that teenagers consider to be a problem, premarital sex relations ranked number one. Here are the things teenagers are concerned about:

1. Premarital relations – 99 percent
2. Drug abuse – 85 percent
3. Alcoholism – 71 percent
4. Suicide – 67 percent
5. Teenage pregnancy – 44 percent
6. Teenage pornography and prostitution – 15 percent.[11]

FALSE PROMISES

For decades, Planned Parenthood and other "family planning" agencies have promised the American public that the crisis of teenage pregnancies, abortions, and sexually transmitted diseases would ease or cease if young people were thoroughly educated about their sexuality, given contraceptive methods and devices, and encouraged to develop sexual practices that were "right for them."

But it would appear that the crisis has escalated, largely as a result of such education—there are now far more pregnancies, abortions, and major epidemics of sexually transmitted diseases than ever before. Proponents claim that the reason for this is a continued *shortage* of comprehensive sex education programs. But this is false. "Different studies produce different figures, but they all confirm that sex education is common across the country. . . . Numerous studies confirm the prevalence, not shortage, of sex education courses in the United States. This finding should cast serious doubt on the [Planned Parenthood subsidiary] Guttmacher Institute's claim that the teen pregnancy rate is due to a lack of programs in the schools."[12]

The reason that so-called comprehensive sex education has failed our children—unfortunately, at their expense—is because many sex educators (1) do not understand the problem and, therefore, (2) propose wrong solutions. Modern sex education is not only a failure, it can be harmful to children in a number of ways.

In fact, it can be demonstrated demographically that wherever "comprehensive sex education programs" exist, the rates of teenage sex activity, pregnancy, abortion, and sexually transmitted diseases continue to mount. But in those districts promoting abstinence, parental involvement, and education concerning the consequences of promiscuity, there is a significant reduction in these four crisis areas. This is documented by Josh McDowell (*The Myths of Sex Education*), Dinah Richards (*Has Sex Education Failed Our Teenagers?: A Research Report*), the research of Jim Sedlak, national director of Stop Planned Parenthood, Brad Hayton (*No Protection: The Failure of Condom-Based Sex Education*), and the research of professor Jacqueline Kasun of San Jose State University, to name a few (see chap. 9).[13]

In February 1992, coauthor John Weldon told a leading representative of Planned Parenthood on national television that studies had confirmed the problems of comprehensive sex education. Her response was only a flat denial that this was true (see chap. 8). She claimed that Planned Parenthood was essential to the nation's health.*

What is so tragic is that we have abandoned our own children to sexual promiscuity in the guise of helping them "handle" their sexuality. But teenagers don't want sex; they want values and meaning in their lives. They want love. In fact, a study conducted in the junior high schools of a major American city revealed that 67 percent of kids said their greatest need in sex education was not the "comprehensive sex education" of Planned Parenthood, but rather learning how to say no to sexual pressure.[14] Even teens can recognize that sexual intimacy is often too powerful for adolescents to handle responsibly—why many sex educators can't seem to understand this is a bit of a mystery.

Susan is a good example. Although Susan was raised in a Christian home and understood the importance of not becoming romantically involved with unbelievers, she fell into the wrong crowd and began dating a young man with whom she soon fell in love.

Susan intuitively knew that she was not ready for sexual activity, but because of her love for this man, she gave in to his continual encouragements to "show her love" for him. Once she had given in, her boyfriend abandoned her, apparently satisfied with his conquest. But Susan was crushed; she felt used and betrayed. It took her several months of counseling and almost a year to heal from the consequences of a single, brief, sexual encounter. "I wish I had known," she said. "I knew I wasn't ready, but I couldn't deal with the intimidation of my sex ed class."

TEEN PROMISCUITY

Teenagers have enough problems today without being encouraged into early sexual activity. Various studies, including one by the U.S. Surgeon General, reveal that many of the nation's teenagers and twenty-three million college students are now drug and alcohol abusers because their lives lack meaning and purpose. Because there is so

---

* To understand how dangerous Planned Parenthood is to the nation's health, see Robert Marshall and Charles Donovan, *Blessed Are the Barren: The Social Policy of Planned Parenthood* (San Francisco: Ignatius, 1991), and George Grant, *Grand Illusion: The Legacy of Planned Parenthood* (Nashville: Wolgemuth & Hyatt, 1988).

little faith in the future, it is also easy for them to "live for today" in terms of physical or sensual gratification. Unfortunately, this only compounds their problems. For example, Brandon told us how he felt about life as a teenager: "Life is so boring. So I've found my own excitement. I don't have a lot of money, but sex is a cheap thrill that doesn't cost anything and can be done anywhere. It is easy to find a girl who is willing. Life is so meaningless anyway, why not?" Brandon never knew that Shirley, one of his "cheap thrills," would later kill herself as a result of his sexual abuse. Or that he would spend twenty years in jail upon conviction of rape.

Teenagers rarely see the consequences of actions that are done in a moment of passion or misguided love. As Mary, a fifteen-year-old girl recalls, "I had no idea what the cost would be. But it took losing my virginity at a very young age, my self-respect, my fertility, bringing ruin to another person's marriage, acquiring an incurable disease, much guilt, and a year and a half of distrusting men before I realized that sex is not something that can be entered into lightly."

On the TV special "C. Everett Koop, M.D., Listening to Teenagers,"[15] the former Surgeon General commented, "Teenagers are walking through a mine field." He noted that most teens have little or no self-esteem, and this leads to drugs, alcohol abuse, and sexual promiscuity. It was startling to hear him say that almost 50 percent of teenagers suffer from depression severe enough to require treatment. Home problems, grade problems, relationship problems, and parental drug and alcohol abuse are some of the causes.

He also emphasized that what adolescents *choose* to do is what puts them at risk. For example, teens can no longer afford to not worry about AIDS (Acquired Immune Deficiency Syndrome), because teenage infection rates are increasing dramatically. Yet more than 50 percent have had sex by eighteen, and every year one in ten teenage girls becomes pregnant. Further, 50 percent of teenagers drink, and one in three is a heavy drinker; thousands die each year in alcohol-induced car accidents—and there are millions of homeless teenagers. Thousands more commit suicide—a "last resort" that is surprisingly not infrequently linked to premarital sexual intercourse (see chap. 10).

What is the solution? Dr. Koop emphasized that "communication is the first step in health care" and that sometimes the right words are better than a doctor's prescription. He noted that lack of communication between parents and teens is the greatest problem we face.

Josh McDowell, who has given more than eighteen thousand talks to more than eight million students and faculty at more than a thousand universities and high schools in seventy-two countries have outlined both the problem and the solution in *The Myths of Sex Education.*

He observes that almost all teenagers and college students have two basic fears—that they will never be loved and that they will never be able to love. As McDowell points out, "One out of every two marriages ends in divorce, and many of the couples who remain married model hatred, distrust or apathy instead of love. No wonder so many kids today are unable to develop close, intimate relationships."[16]

When parents don't show love to their children, those children may search for love elsewhere. One questionnaire among a thousand high school students revealed that 50 percent were uncertain that their parents loved them.[17] McDowell explains: "Fathers are often worse offenders than mothers in failing to communicate love. . . . I truly believe that lots of hugs between fathers and their teen daughters would do more to stop the teen pregnancy epidemic than any other single factor."[18]

In discussing the reasons that children become sexually involved, McDowell further reveals,

> If I had to give one reason, I would say [they] get sexually involved in search of a father's love. . . . We don't have a teenage sexual crisis—we have a teenage/parental relationship crisis. Teens are looking for intimacy from those who love them, particularly their fathers. When they don't find it there, they turn to sexual activity to get it. . . . Our kids don't want sex as much as they want to be loved. It's as true for sons as it is for daughters. . . . They want someone who cares, who will listen and who will talk to them, and they want it to start with their fathers. This is the heartache of the broken home, whether through a legal divorce, an "emotional divorce" between parents and their children, or simply a lack of love and communication. Kids who are not loved at home will look for love in all the wrong places.[19]

It can't be denied that need for love and intimacy is one of the deepest needs we experience. Unfortunately, this is something that liberal sex education, thinking it is working on behalf of teens, continues to deny them by promoting the very promiscuity and personal insecurity it seeks to prevent.

Fathers and mothers need to learn not only how to express love to their children, but they also need to know the facts concerning the current social situation in which their children are being reared and educated by society. If the sexual epidemic is a search for love, and parents meet their children's need for love, coupled with a common sense, abstinence-based presentation of sex education, then the current tragedy can be halted.

2

Safer Sex: How Safe Is It?

What They're Teaching Our Kids

"Mike" was a well-known first baseman for a major league ball club. Although he had made a commitment to Christ at a young age, he discovered that becoming a baseball superstar in high school, college, and professional sports brought its own unique set of challenges, including how to deal with his increasingly worldly lifestyle. Mike also discovered that many women were freely willing to give themselves to him. Although he was able to handle this pressure in high school and college, once he became a national superstar he found it almost impossible to resist the constant attentions of beautiful women. He began to enjoy the adulation of these women and didn't even care that many of them wanted to have sex with him only as a "trophy."

When Mike was in high school and college, AIDS did not exist. But AIDS is now a concern, and, once Mike decided that he was going to take advantage of all the beautiful women in his life, he knew he had better learn how to practice "safe sex."

When we met Mike, he was at the peak of his career. We had a discussion about biblical morality and the consequences of sexual promiscuity. Mike replied that he didn't care what the Bible taught.

In the next several years Mike had sex with scores of women, convinced that he was not at risk because he practiced safe sex. Even though he sometimes found it difficult to abide by his own rules, he felt that the odds of getting AIDS were almost nonexistent.

But not only did Mike eventually get herpes, clamydia, gonorrhea, and syphilis, he is now being tested for probable exposure to AIDS.

He exists in emotional misery, and his career is in jeopardy. Still a young man, he wonders, *What will I do if I test positive?*

A CONTRADICTION OF TERMS

Many voices in society are telling teenagers and almost everyone else that they can have safe sex. Planned Parenthood, Hugh Hefner and founders of various "adult" magazines, the increasingly powerful political lobby of the homosexual/lesbian community, certain feminists, popular talk-show hosts such as Phil Donohue, as well as Dr. Ruth and other so-called sex authorities are only a few. But consider the following dictionary definitions of *safe*:

The Oxford American Dictionary—"**1.** free from risk or danger, not dangerous. **2.** providing security or protection."

Webster's 20th International Dictionary—"**1.** free from harm, injury or risk; no longer threatened by danger or injury."

The Macmillan Dictionary for Students—"**3.** affording security, protection; **4.** involving no risk, uncertainty or danger of failure, mishap or error."

Given the above definitions and the serious risks involved in any casual sexual intercourse today, it should be obvious that "safe sex" is a contradiction of terms (see chaps. 3, 5, 6, 11). At least the more responsible commentators now refer to "safer sex"—indicating that they realize there may be a few leaks in things other than condoms. But anyone with a pencil and paper can take a few minutes to calculate that, given the following facts, the world is headed for a major health disaster:

1. *"Safe sex" isn't safe; even if it were, people aren't changing their sexual attitudes or behavior.*[1] Most people don't practice safe sex in spite of hundreds of millions of dollars spent on educational campaigns. Further, people frequently lie to their partners about their sexual history and even whether they are currently infected with AIDS or other STDs.[2] According to ABC "AIDs Update," August 10, 1991, many people cannot trust what others say about their sexual lives—40 percent of men and 10 percent of women lied about past risky sexual behavior; further, 20 percent of men said they had been tested for HIV when they had not.

2. *The common figure is that some ten million people worldwide are infected with HIV (Human Immunodeficiency Virus). But a more*

realistic figure may be fifty million. HIV mutation rates and mode of transmission uncertainty mean that the actual number of infected could be much higher. No one knows. Five to ten years may pass before symptoms appear in some infected persons, and in spite of testing, the disease is sometimes undetectable for up to fourteen months.[3] Thus, millions of people around the world already have the disease without knowing it, and they are spreading it to others. Also, many who know they are infected have no intention of changing their sex life simply because it might harm someone else. Homosexuals, prostitutes, and drug users—the principal current carriers in America—may not be so concerned about safe sex if most of them suspect they are already infected.

For years cigarette manufacturers promised that smoking did not cause cancer. Smoking was a "safe" practice. It wasn't until lung cancer reached immense proportions that society finally realized that smoking was no laughing matter and certainly not safe on the basis of the assurances of vested interests.

Likewise, for years, those who used drugs such as marijuana and cocaine were promised by others that these drugs were "safe and harmless." Today we have a five-year-old war on drugs that has spent billions and hardly won a single battle: among adults, overall, drug use is up in every category.[4]

Today we are told that sex can be safe. Basketball superstar Magic Johnson accepted a position with the President's Commission on AIDS because he was such a fine role model for youth. But can a man who contracts AIDS because of his sexual immorality be considered a role model to youth concerning sexual responsibility? Wilt Chamberlain, another role model, once boasted that he had had sex with more than twenty thousand women! What messages are we sending our kids when we encourage our children to idolize such figures?

According to "NBC Evening News" on November 18, 1991, since Magic Johnson's announcement that he had AIDS hardly anyone had changed his or her behavior and was now practicing safe sex. Consider some characteristic comments of those interviewed: "It's just passion." "There's no escaping it." "You live for the moment." "Sex is a natural act." These responses by teens and collegians are those commonly heard throughout the country in schools, bars, and middle-class homes. NBC concluded that most people are listening to their hormones and continuing to freely engage in sex rather than listen to the warnings that they might die.

As Jerry, a sophomore college student, told us, "The social pressure I feel to have sex and my own need for love outweigh the possible consequences. If I die, I die. That's what part of me says. The other part hopes I don't hurt someone I love—or give them AIDS. I know I am sexually active, and I know there are risks. I also know I will never be tested because I just couldn't bear the thought of knowing that I was going to die. When I think about it, it's a terrible thing to be having sex and never knowing whether you have exposed yourself to AIDS. You honestly don't want anyone else to die, but your own insecurities and needs sometimes outweigh the possible risks to other people. So, I try not to think about it."

Until recently it seems that the only admonitions against premarital sex were to be found in the Bible. But now alarms are heard everywhere. Whether or not they are heeded, no one can deny the wisdom of what God spoke two thousand years ago:

> Let us behave decently, as in the daytime, not in orgies and drunkenness, not in sexual immorality and debauchery, not in dissension and jealousy. (Romans 13:13)

> The body is not meant for sexual immorality, but for the Lord, and the Lord for the body. . . . Flee from sexual immorality. All other sins a man commits are outside his body, but he who sins sexually sins against his own body. Do you not know that your body is a temple of the Holy Spirit, who is in you, whom you have received from God? You are not your own; you were bought at a price. Therefore, honor God with your body. (1 Corinthians 6:13, 18–20)

> But among you there must not be even a hint of sexual immorality, or of any kind of impurity, or of greed, because these are improper for God's holy people. (Ephesians 5:3)

> Put to death, therefore, whatever belongs to your earthly nature: sexual immorality, impurity, lust, evil desires and greed, which is idolatry. Because of these, the wrath of God is coming. (Colossians 3:5–6)

> It is God's will that you should be sanctified: that you should avoid sexual immorality; that each of you should learn to control his own body in a way that is holy and honorable, not in passionate lust like the heathen, who do not know God; and that in this matter no one should wrong his brother or take advantage of him. The Lord will punish men for all such sins, as we have already told you and warned you. For God did not call us to be impure, but to live a holy life. Therefore, he who rejects this instruction does not reject man but God, who gives you his Holy Spirit. (1 Thessalonians 4:3–8)

STILL IN A MESS

Oxford scholar C. S. Lewis revealed the irony of our situation:

> Perversions of the sex instinct are numerous, hard to cure, and frightful. I am sorry to have to go into all these details, but I must. The reason why I must is that you and I, for the last twenty years, have been fed all day long on good solid lies about sex. We have been told, until one is sick of hearing it, that sexual desire is in the same state as any of our other natural desires and that if only we abandon the silly old Victorian idea of hushing it up, everything in the garden will be lovely. It is not true. The moment you look at the facts, and away from the propaganda, you see that it is not.
> They tell you sex has become a mess because it was hushed up. But for the last twenty years it has not been hushed up. It has been chattered about all day long. Yet it is still in a mess. If hushing up had been the cause of the trouble, ventilation would have set it right. But it has not. I think it is the other way round. I think the human race originally hushed it up because it had become such a mess.[5]

Ironically, the birth of AIDS and fifty other sexually transmitted diseases suggests it won't be long before we again face a "mess"—this time of unparalleled proportions.

In the last thirty years we have increasingly removed God and absolute moral values from our national culture. Since then we have experienced a dramatic rise in divorce rate, illegal drug use, crime, child abuse reports, suicide levels, educational decline, political corruption, teenage pregnancies, economic dislocations, sexually transmitted diseases, pornography, abortion, and many other social ills.

Teaching Safer Sex is a teaching manual put out by Planned Parenthood of Bergen County (New Jersey). The authors of the manual are well aware of the risks of sexual activity today: "Young people are at high risk for all sexually transmitted diseases. Every year, one out of seven 15 to 24-year-olds becomes infected with an STD. And there is evidence that adolescents may be one of the next high risk groups for HIV infection."[6] Yet this manual claims that it is "dangerous" to teach abstinence as the only acceptable option—even while it admits that increased sexual information does not guarantee a change in behavior. Unfortunately, the major message of this teaching aid is an encouragement for kids to have sexual intercourse.

The authors of *Teaching Safer Sex* explain why they wrote a text on safe sex:

> In an age of AIDS, "safer sex" must become the norm, . . . [yet] recent research indicates that although most young people *know the basic facts* about HIV transmission and how to avoid contracting the virus, they are *not yet changing high risk behaviors*. . . . Groups that have historically opposed sex education are using the AIDS crisis to demand that abstinence until marriage be taught as the only acceptable option. This is dangerous. . . . To be effective, prevention education must be realistic.[7] (Italics added).

When the manual itself confesses that "statistics show that 50 percent of the population contracts an STD by the time they are twenty-four,"[8] one can only wonder who is being "realistic" and why they reject an abstinence-only approach. Fifty percent of the population is an incredibly large figure. Looking at all the widespread consequences of sexual permissiveness in our society today, is abstinence only really a "dangerous" approach—or is it the other way around?

As a reflection of current trends, the manual gives specific instruction in how to teach children "safe" intercourse. It also tells them that "outercourse" may be better for them than intercourse. Thus, "participants will recognize the importance of 'outercouse' as a safer sex option. . . . Most of the pleasures of intercourse are possible and much more safe, without intercourse. . . . A commitment to 'outercourse' provides couples with the opportunity to enjoy their sexuality in many new ways, ways that avoid most risks of disease transmission as well as the risk of an unwanted pregnancy."[9]

Children are encouraged to have group discussions on suggesting various forms of outercourse. "A list may include: . . . body massage, bathing together, masturbation, mutual masturbation, sensuous feeding, fantasizing, watching erotic movies, reading erotic books and magazines."[10]

Participants are to be divided into pairs or small groups. They are asked to write a slogan advertising the benefits of outercourse, printing it on construction paper and taping it to the wall. Sample slogans are offered by the teacher to encourage the students. For example, "Outercourse is in." "Outercourse? Of course!" "People do it every night—outercourse is delight without fright." "Outercourse. The choice of a safe generation." "Outercourse and you, perfect together."[11]

Further, "participants will internalize the concept of sexual safety by becoming advocates for it." And, "participants become advocates for the very behaviors that will enhance their own safety."[12]

But how many kids who are explicitly instructed in techniques of outercourse—and encouraged to practice it—can long avoid progressing to intercourse? Is outercourse instruction realistic—or is it just fueling the fire?

In the section on condoms titled "Worksheet: Using Condoms" the child is instructed to "keep condoms handy so they can be used every time you have intercourse."[13] "If you have never used a condom, or don't feel comfortable using one, you can practice putting a condom on a banana, cucumber or dildo. Men who masturbate can practice on themselves."[14] In addition, students are encouraged to discover where they can buy condoms in their local communities and evaluate the different brands and types of condoms sold.[15]

In another lesson, students are told how to talk to potential sex partners. "Participants will rehearse talking with a partner about sex in a variety of situations."[16] (See addendum for further examples.)

If texts such as these are now widely distributed around the country, is it any wonder we face a crisis?

In conclusion, if it is established that "safer sex" really isn't safe, then manuals such as this that actively encourage young people to engage in intercourse and "outercourse" are not in their best interests. If, as taxpayers, parents do not want their money being spent to teach their children information such as this, they should let this be known to both their political representatives and their local Planned Parenthood/school board.

ADDENDUM:
MORE ABOUT *TEACHING SAFER SEX*

Teaching Safer Sex also encourages homosexuality. The instructor is told the following: "References to couples, whether visual or verbal, will include same sex and opposite sex partners. References to sex will include sex between same sex partners unless the lesson specifies vaginal intercourse or risk of pregnancy."[17] The manual further presents the Kinsey falsehood concerning a 10 percent occurrence of homosexuality in the population: "Given the fact that one in ten people are gay or lesbian, it is important that safer sex education not ignore homosexual young people who are likely to be present in any audience."[18] The teacher is even asked to distribute a "Worksheet: On Being Gay—a Bibliography for Young People" containing more than twenty books promoting homosexuality. The Hetrick-Martin Institute (formerly the Institute for the Protection of Gay and Lesbian Youth) is recommended for further information and resources.[19]

In "A Workshop for High Risk Use" the teacher is told to introduce the lesson by saying this class is "about sex in the age of AIDS and how it can still be safe and responsible, erotic and fun. Expect some laughter and joking and be ready to join in."[20] Under point four we find the following:

> 4. Proper condom use. Put up another sheet of newsprint with the title, "HOW TO USE A CONDOM." Ask the students to list all the steps in sequence. If someone calls out a step that should come later, say, "yes, but what should come before that?" Here is a list of the proper steps. Write them down in the language used by the young people.
>   a. Open the condom package (careful not to tear the condom!).
>   b. Get an erection.
>   c. Rub a small dab of lubricant (K–Y or other water-soluable lub) on tip of penis (increases sensitivity and adhesion).
>   d. Keep air out of reservoir tip (can lead to busting).
>   e. Roll it down good—be erotic about it.
>   f. Put lots of lubricant on outside of condom (use unlubricated condoms for oral sex).
>   g. Do it!
>   h. Just before orgasm, pull out with the condom on.
>   i. If you have had an orgasm without pulling out beforehand, grip end of condom and pull out before penis goes limp.
> 5. Demystifying condoms. Hand out condoms to everyone, ask them to open the package carefully, and then let them play with them. They can taste them, stretch them, blow them up, or try to tear them. They will see how durable the condom is. . . .
> 6. Using condoms. Hand out the bananas (or zucchini or cucumbers). Show them the K–Y and Vaseline and ask them which lubricant to use and why. . . . Now have the students practice putting the condoms on properly, following all the steps that they had listed before. If you don't have bananas or the like for everyone, have two clients demonstrate how to use the condom by putting one on a dildo, or the condom can be rolled down on two fingers of one hand. (Male clients who masturbate can be encouraged to try out a condom at home when doing so).[21]

Also described is the "Safety Dance: Safer Sex Dance Party," which is labeled as possibly not being appropriate for high school situations, although it is used in them and even assigned as homework.[22] Besides a condom relay race and "breaking the condom pinata at midnight," there is also the "putting on the condom" role-playing where the participants arrange themselves in a line or circle according to how they think a condom is used. "Acting out the steps can increase the fun of this activity." Among the twenty-four steps listed from the first (physical attraction) to the last (deciding where to throw away the used condom) are: "Think about having sex," "Talk about having sex," "Decide to use a condom," "Pool money," "Decide what kind to buy," "Meet your lover," "Decide to have sex," "Roll condom down penis," and "Intercourse."[23]

The High Risk of Condoms

Are They Enough Protection?

Bill and Sandy were in love and soon to be engaged. After discussing the issue of having sex together, they decided that they wanted to begin a sexual relationship as a way to "test their compatibility" before engagement. They were also a little frightened. Both Bill and Sandy had been involved in several sexual relationships with other people before falling in love. They realized the possibility might exist that they had an undiagnosed, latent STD or had possibly been exposed to the AIDS virus.

Bill and Sandy concluded that, even though they didn't like the idea, the most responsible thing to do would be for Bill to use a condom. But they discovered they didn't like it at all; it detracted from the spontaneity, joy, and feeling of their sexual relationship.

Although they did their best to practice safe sex, they found that they were successful only about 20 percent of the time. In the end, they concluded that they would simply take the risk and hope that neither of them had been exposed in the past. Bill told us, "Well, what can you do? Safe sex is just too inconvenient and artificial. Besides, I'm feeling fine and in good health, and the chances are good I'm clean."

Even though both Sandy and Bill could have visited a health clinic to be tested for the major STDs, neither of them felt comfortable with the idea. As it turns out, Bill lied to his girlfriend. He told her that he had less than five relationships with other women before meeting her. In fact, he had had more than twenty. He decided not to tell the truth because he couldn't bear the possibility of losing the one that he finally loved. So he kept his past a secret and hoped for the best. It was easy to convince himself that things were OK because AIDS was primarily a disease of gays and drug users.

But Bill should have told the truth. Today, he has been diagnosed as HIV positive and has no idea how he is going to tell Sandy. He hopes desperately that he has not infected her. For her part, she is curious as to his recent dogmatic demand that he always use a condom.

Bill is in torment, and Sandy is confused. She suspects something but, right now, is also frightened to pursue the matter for fear of what it might do to their relationship or what it might mean to her future. Bill has no idea what to do.

Today, "condoms" and "safe sex" are almost synonymous. But truly safe sex can be had only through permanent monogamy in which you are 100 percent certain that your partner is uninfected—a rare piece of knowledge today. Condoms may *reduce* the risk of AIDS and some other STDs, but they do not *prevent* them. Nor should condoms be considered society's solution to AIDS or other STD transmission.

Nevertheless, according to a Gallup Poll released August 27, 1992, 68 percent of adults responding approved of condom distribution in their local public schools. (Cities already having school-based condom availability programs include Los Angles, Chicago, Philadelphia, New York, Baltimore, Portland, and Miami.) This figure is surprisingly high, but if such a figure is accurate, it underscores the basic problem we are concerned about in this book: permissive attitudes toward sexuality in general and a lack of understanding the real issues involved.

WHY CONDOMS FAIL

The problem with condoms is threefold: (1) they are infrequently used because many think they don't feel good; (2) even when the intent to use is present, they are often not used because of the passionate nature of the sex act; and (3) when they are used, they may be used improperly as a result of drugs or alcohol, and even in the best of circumstances they can break, leak, or slip. In other words, the effectiveness of condoms is directly proportional to the frequency of condom use and the failure rate of the condom itself.

But even 100 percent usage with a 0 percent failure rate will not prevent transmission of the AIDS virus because the virus may simply go through the condom (see below). Regardless, most people just don't like condoms. Incredibly, a June 1990 study of teenagers in San Francisco revealed that almost half thought that "sex without condoms is worth the risk of AIDS."[1]

Though condom use is better than no condom use, again, no one should consider it safe. According to McDowell, "The Department of Health and Human Services reports: 'one of every five batches of condoms tested in a government inspection program over the last four months failed to meet minimum standards for leaks.'"[2]

Further, according to *Consumer Reports* (March 1989), FDA inspectors "checked more than 150,000 samples from lots representing 120 million condoms. The agents had to reject about one lot in ten of domestic condoms because too many leaked. Imports turned out to be worse—one in five lots was rejected." Other studies indicate a lower leakage rate of 1 percent among U.S. condoms but still as high as 20 percent among foreign products.[3] Regardless, one study revealed that the overall condom rupture rate was 5 percent, and they concluded, "Truly safe sex with an HIV-positive partner using condoms is a dangerous illusion."[4]

The fact that condoms can break, leak, and slip is why condoms are not safe when it comes to AIDS or other sexually transmitted diseases. In laboratory tests, four of the most popular brands allowed the AIDS virus to escape.[5] Although latex condoms are more effective in blocking the AIDS virus, many people continue to use the more expensive lambskin condoms because they feel better. The AIDS virus can more easily pass through them because it is some 450 times smaller than a single sperm. *Consumer Reports* observes that scanning the membranes of lambskin condoms under an electron microscope showed that the lattice work making up the condom skins revealed occasional pores up to 1.5 microns. This size pore is smaller than a sperm, white blood cell, or even some gonorrhea bacteria. But it is ten times the size of the AIDS virus and more than twenty-five times the size of the hepatitis-B virus, another major scourge of sexually related activity.[6]

Steve and Mary were a couple who prided themselves on a responsible approach to sexual intercourse. They kept informed on the latest data concerning the spread of major STDs, including AIDS. Before they entered into a sexual relationship, they promised each other that they would commit themselves to a 100 percent monogamous relationship and the careful use of only latex condoms. Everything they had read had told them that latex condoms prevented HIV infection—which, of course, was the last thing they wanted to deal with. Steve and Mary truly believed that they were impervious to HIV infection and that they were judiciously engaging in truly safe sex.

But has research indisputably proven that even latex condoms invariably act as a barrier against the AIDS virus? No. Laboratory tests have indicated that they are "more impermeable to HIV in the laboratory" than natural membrane condoms, but not 100 percent impermeable.[7] That is one reason that, at best, "the actual effectiveness of condom use in the prevention of HIV transmission has been difficult to assess."[8]

In a two-year study among heterosexuals in general, condom failure for HIV transmission ranged from 17 to 30 percent—that's a significant probability of infection. How can that be considered safe?[9] "Researchers studied AIDS transmission among spouses in which one partner was infected with the virus. The results showed that the rate of transmission between couples using condoms was 17 percent over a relatively short time (eighteen months)."[10]

The Washington, D. C., based organization Americans for a Sound AIDS/HIV Policy comments, "Regarding the use of condoms as a preventative measure, scientific studies now make it clear that condoms cannot guarantee safety. The failure rates of condoms in protecting against unwanted pregnancies, syphilis, gonnorhea, and genital herpes, as well as HIV infection, vary from 5 percent to 30 percent."[11]

A Department of Health and Human Services Task Force offered the following sobering conclusion that "there are no clinical (human trial) data to support the value of condoms" in preventing the spread of a wide range of sexually transmitted diseases, including AIDS, herpes, syphilis, and hepatitis-B.[12]

Dr. Nicholas Fiumara, then director of the Massachusetts Department of Public Health, revealed that, all things considered, condoms are often ineffective against both gonorrhea and syphilis: "In summary, then, its ineffectiveness makes the condom useless as a prophylactic against gonorrhea, and even under ideal conditions against syphilis."[13] For example, "The condom is effective against gonorrhea provided there is no preliminary sex play, the condom is intact before use, the condom is put on correctly, and the condom is taken off correctly. However, the male population has never been able to fulfill the very first requisite."[14]

Among the homosexual population, one Pittsburgh study revealed that in anal sex 15 percent of the condoms slipped off and 11 percent ruptured.[15] Another study indicated that condom failure could be as high as 50 percent.[16] Perhaps this and other studies are why a U.S. Public Health and Human Services Task Force recently warned, "The risk of condom failure in anal intercourse is so high that the practice should be avoided entirely—with condoms or without."[17]

Even though Harry and Sam had been committed lovers for over a year, neither one really trusted the other to remain absolutely faithful. They had done their best to use condoms, but found the practice difficult to maintain. As they continued homosexual practices, they discovered they were becoming increasingly careless. As the depressing news over AIDS continued to mount, their corresponding resignation to their apparent "fate" overtook the relationship. Indeed, they found such resignation everywhere they went in the gay community. Harry told us, "Most active gays have resigned themselves to being infected. So have we. So, let the good times roll."

Today, both Harry and Sam remain asymptomatic, but they have each taken several additional lovers while maintaining their "nuclear" relationship with one another. Both have discussed this openly, and they have agreed. Sam and Harry are resigned to the fact that most homosexuals are already infected—and that life is short anyway.

Clarence and Studs find themselves in a similar situation. They know that the risks of homosexual behavior are still high even with condom use and have decided that the hassle is just not worth it. After attempting safe sex, they now engage in sex in any manner they wish. They live for the pure enjoyment of physical gratification just as they did before. Both are convinced that if they are not yet HIV positive, they will be—and that nothing can be done to stop it.

Thus, even with safe sex —i.e., the use of condoms—the likelihood is that AIDS will continue to spread among both the homosexual and heterosexual population. That is why authorities are increasingly warning that equating condom use with safety in sexual behavior is a dangerously false premise. Dr. Robert Redfield is the army AIDS specialist at the Department of Retroviral Research, Walter Reed Army Institute of Research, who recently made discoveries in AIDS vaccine therapy (called GP160). He emphasizes, "Condoms are *not* safe. They're dangerous. Sex with a condom with an infected person is not protected [sex]. It's very *unprotected* [sex]. It's very, very dangerous."[18]

Redfield, who is an expert on science, HIV, and public policy is "strongly against" the condom message even though he initially supported it. The principal reason is that condoms fail too often. He says, "The truth is, condoms are not an appropriate medical or public health solution to this epidemic. It is a quick-fix strategy. It's not going to work, and the price of this strategy is that we are losing precious time to re-educate, train and equip our young people on how to avoid becoming a statistic in the AIDS epidemic. It's *not* by wearing condoms. It's by teaching them sexual integrity and how to use the gift of human sexuality as it was meant to be used."[19]

Dr. Harold Jaffee, chief of epidemiology for the Centers for Disease Control in Atlanta, argues that it is morally wrong to tell people that they can do whatever they want as long as they wear a condom. Referring to AIDS, he says, "It is just too dangerous a disease to say that."[20] Infectious disease specialist Robert C. Noble warns, "Passing out condoms to teenagers is like issuing them squirt guns for a four alarm blaze."[21]

Theresa Crenshaw, M.D., past president of the American Association of Sex Educators, Counselors and Therapists, and a member of the Presidential AIDS Commission, says that equating condom use with safe sex "is, in fact, playing Russian roulette. A lot of people will die in this dangerous game."[22]

Lieutenant Colonel Donald Burke is a graduate of the Harvard Medical School and Director of the Department of Retroviral Research, Walter Reed Army Institute of Research, in Washington, D.C. He is also the originator of the army's HIV screening program and an expert on HIV public health policy. He comments, "Condom usage has been promoted as one of the cornerstones of HIV epidemic control, but there are some problems with that strategy. One of the problems [is that] it implies the number of partners you have really doesn't matter; you can go ahead and have an unlimited number of sexual partners—and that protection in the form of a condom will interrupt transmission. Although condoms are effective to *some* degree, they are not entirely effective. . . . [With] a fatal communicable disease, how can we afford that risk?"[23]

Dr. Malcolm Potts, president of Family Health International and one of the inventors of condoms lubricated with spermicides, confesses that no one can tell people how much protection condoms give and that encouraging a person who engages in high-risk behavior to use a condom "is like telling someone who is driving drunk to use a seat belt."[24]

Perhaps the most compelling argument against the "condoms as safe sex" approach is the fact that not a single medical expert in the world would knowingly proceed to have intercourse with an AIDS-infected person using a condom—in the supposition that that would protect him or her from AIDS.

Consider the irony here. The centerpiece of the current medical public health message is the use of condoms to prevent HIV infection. But if both partners aren't infected, condoms play no role in prevention. The same is true if both partners are infected. The only preventative role condoms play is when one partner is infected and another isn't. Yet, *medically* speaking, no M.D. anywhere would encourage an uninfected person to have sex with an infected person merely because he used a condom. In other words, the medical pillar for preventing HIV infection is something so dangerous no doctor would ever recommend it to anyone![25]

RISK REDUCTION OR RISK ELIMINATION?

It seems clear that the present policy of risk *reduction* is only helping to *spread* sexually transmitted diseases, including AIDS. National policy must be changed to a philosophy of risk *elimination*—abstinence and life-long monogamy with an uninfected partner. As an article in the *New England Journal of Medicine* recently noted, "Reducing risky sex rather than eliminating it is like incompletely immunizing a population—there is little benefit to the individual or the community."[26] The bottom line is that by definition so-called risk reduction accepts a certain rate of death. Risk elimination does not—abstinence does not include the sentence of death.

As a society, we have the choice of encouraging a death index or of rejecting the concept entirely. Since it is we and our children who are at risk, what is the only sane choice?[27]

But worse still, it appears that the entire safe sex campaign may emerge as a red herring because, as noted, most people—homosexuals and heterosexuals alike—simply refuse to practice safe sex. According to Mindy Fullilove, M.D., of the HIV Center for Clinical and Behavioral Studies at Columbia University, even in 1992, most heterosexual men and women still do not perceive themselves to be at risk.[28]

John and Melinda are typical examples. They continue to believe that AIDS is primarily a homosexual disease and that infection rates among heterosexuals are so small as to be meaningless. They are more concerned about herpes and other incurable STDs than about HIV. John and his fiancée believe that AIDS will never become a heterosexual problem, and therefore safer sex isn't even an issue.

But both have told us that even if AIDS were to dramatically increase among heterosexuals they would continue to engage in *un*safe sex simply because sex is such an important part of their lives—and, anyway, everything in life carries some degree of risk.

Melinda explained, "Look, I distrust marriage, I don't want kids and life is meaningless anyway. Enjoy what you can and don't worry about what you can't control." John and Melinda are not unique.

A study of 16,632 women in Pennsylvania revealed that only 13 percent used condoms while 72 percent *never* used condoms even with casual partners.[29]

The National Education Association's guide for teachers *The Facts About AIDS*, part of their massive condom campaign, states, "Health education that relies only on the transmission of information is ineffective. Behavioral change results only when information is supported by shared community values that are powerfully conveyed."[30]

Consider that a National Institute of Health study of almost five thousand gay and bi-sexual men revealed that more than 50 percent still practiced receptive anal sex and that more than two-thirds did not use condoms.[31]

Other studies indicate similar results. Most homosexual men who continue to engage in unprotected anal sex (1) have had knowledge of safe sex techniques, (2) agree that condoms could reduce the spread of AIDS, and (3) identified anal sex as the highest-risk category for AIDS. Regardless, the majority indicated that they "never" or "hardly ever" used condoms during anal intercourse and that their partners "never" or "hardly ever" did. The majority also reported multiple sexual partners within the last six months. Worse still, almost one-fourth reported that half or more of their sexual partners were anonymous.[32]

Finally, numerous collegiate studies indicate that knowledge of safe sex practices and AIDS prevention is high, but many or most students have not altered their sexual habits. For example, a survey of 5,500 Canadian college students revealed that in spite of a high level of awareness about the dangers of AIDS, less than 16 percent of the women always had their partners use condoms. A study at the University of Florida showed that only 20 percent of students always used condoms.[33]

Today, people are educated on all kinds of dangers—even life threatening ones—and yet continue to practice the same unsafe activities, whether it is not using seat belts, drunk driving, cigarette smoking—or sex. People deny the dangers because they don't want to believe them, and they prefer the convenience or pleasure to the perceived risk. The large gap between education and behavior will probably remain until the majority of the population sees itself at great risk personally.

All this is why condoms should not be considered a safe solution to the spread of AIDS. Nor should a "value free" education that rejects or demeans morality and abstinence be considered a solution.

In conclusion, those who want to risk death should continue their behavior—with or without condoms and safe sex. Those who desire truly safe sex (at least medically) should remember that the only behavior carrying a 100 percent guarantee of safety is abstinence—or lifelong monogamous sex with a person who you are 100 percent certain is not infected with AIDS or anything else.

Abstinence: Is It Really a Dirty Word?

Why the Cultural Elite Thinks So

In their best-selling *Why Wait? What You Need to Know About the Teen Sexuality Crisis,* Josh McDowell and Dick Day provide many illustrations from the lives of teens concerning the problems they face as adolescents and the consequences they encounter for poor decision making in the area of sexuality. Noting that the consequences of premarital sex can be devastating, they cite a young woman who commented, "The reality of pregnancy outside of marriage is scary and lonely. To have premarital sex was my choice one hot June night, forcing many decisions I thought I would never have to make. Those decisions radically changed my life."[1]

Another young woman writes, "The reason I'm writing this is I am alone and confused. My boyfriend kept pursuing me for sex. . . . I had sex with him thinking that I owed it to him. . . . Later when I learned I was pregnant, he blew up, said to get an abortion, and that it was all my fault. So to save my parents heartache and to keep Matt, I had an abortion. Now, Matt has left me."[2]

Literally millions of teenagers across the country are uncertain about how to deal with the sexual pressure they face and are asking for help. It is up to parents and society to help them—or face the consequences.

PREOCCUPATION WITH SEX

The real cause of the nation's sexual pandemic—teenage pregnancy, AIDS, abortion, STDs, and broken lives—largely results from the American preoccupation with sex and the biased and false assumptions about sexuality that permeate society (see chap. 12). These falsehoods have resulted in unworkable "solutions" to the very problems they created. Consider the false assumption that teenagers are going to practice sex and there is nothing anyone can do about it. That is one of the biggest myths being propagated, because 33 to 50 percent of all teenagers are now practicing abstinence. And studies prove that given accurate information and proper encouragement, many sexually active teens will also adopt a lifestyle of abstinence.[3] Abstinence-based sex education works, as many studies now prove.[4]

But aren't many parents equally to blame for the current situation? Has their own sexual behavior communicated wrong sexual attitudes to their children? Even parents with high moral standards have caved in to the sexual permissiveness of the times.

Consider the case of Harold and June who upheld strong moral values and had been married for ten years before Harold entered into an extended mid-life crisis, which began to compromise his convictions. Feeling bored with his marriage and knowing it was wrong to enter into an adulterous relationship, Harold did so anyway in a reckless attempt to prove to himself that he was still attractive to younger women. "I was desperate," he recalls. "Anyway, you see it everywhere—on TV, in the movies, among your friends. I couldn't escape it."

Unknown to him, his wife had also felt an increasing insecurity in their relationship and was already engaging in an extramarital affair in an attempt to find someone who understood her. She too thought she needed to prove to herself that she was still attractive to men.

But soon after their affairs, their marriage relationship began to suffer in unexpected ways. Almost intuitively neither trusted the other. Tempers were short, and problems once easily resolved became major barriers to communication. Things got worse and worse.

The children also knew something was wrong but didn't know what it was or what to do about it. Finally, Harold decided that the stress was too much. He moved out of the house to live with another woman—his former lover. His son and daughter were crushed, but his wife felt the worst pain she had ever experienced.

Ironically, until their initial extramarital affairs, both parents had attempted to instill a moral perspective in their children regarding sexual behavior. They realized that sex was something that would be difficult for children to handle as they entered their teenage years.

But after experiencing sexual infidelity personally, they found it more and more difficult to present moral values to their teenagers. In fact, Harold even decided that his son and daughter were probably going to get sexually involved anyway and there was nothing he could do about it. As a result, he abandoned the dating standards he had set, giving as his only counsel the advice to "make certain no one gets pregnant." Harold eventually divorced his wife, who ended up living with another man.

Several years down the road, the repercussions of the parents' sin had finally worked its way into their children's lives. By seventeen, their son had gotten his girlfriend pregnant (she had an abortion) and their daughter had contracted herpes and PID, which brought sterility.

Almost without realizing it, both parents, who had begun their marriage with the finest of intentions, had let slip away what was truly important in life. They had adopted the values they saw in their culture rather than standing against them. They learned a sad lesson and so had their children: sexual promiscuity can exact a terrible price.

Illicit sex is glamorized in movies, television programs, and magazines. We have accepted it as part of modern life. Peer pressure compounds the problem. Parents who refuse to accept moral absolutes compound it further. Then liberal educators put the final nail in the coffin.

HOW WE TREAT OUR KIDS

Although many Christian parents desire to educate their children biblically, they often fail. For their part, the children often regret it, even though the parents rarely discover this until years later. What a terrible waste! At no time is a person more susceptible to being taught spiritual things than as a child or young adult. Here are statements made by teenagers themselves:

> I wish my parents knew how much I want to become a stronger Christian! Both my parents are Christians, but we don't talk about it much. We all go to church and we pray, and they have taught me well. I just wish we could talk about the Lord more!

> Dad—I love you, and I wish when I was younger we had spent more time together. Although you and Mom are both Christians, I wish you would have been a stronger spiritual influence in my life.

Dad, why did you quit after-dinner devotions after only a week just because we complained that we wanted to play instead? We were only kids!

I think parents need to inform kids about what sex is in the beginning, and also should tell them the Scriptures. When you are young, it is really confusing, because there are so many things you don't know, and you need to have some backup help like the Bible. But I think sometimes parents don't want to talk about it.

I wish my parents knew how much it would have meant to me if our home had been more dedicated to the study of God's word. I wish they would renew their own devotion to each other and to God. I wish my dad would put Christ first in his life. I wish they knew how important these things are to me.

Most teenagers aren't properly educated in sexual matters. They know what comes naturally, but they don't understand God's interpretation of sexual love. They don't know they are doing wrong because they haven't been exposed to the right. They have no religious background or else it isn't a firmly sound background. They are ignorant in a highly promoted subject, thus, they tend to make unwise choices.[5]

In the authors' personal experience, among the saddest circumstances they have encountered are the consequences of Christian parents failing to educate their children spiritually and biblically. Rather than rearing their children to love Jesus above all else and to be committed to Bible study, they have not made Christian education in the home their priority. In the end, they may find they have raised children with worldly standards who, not surprisingly, adopt the world's set of priorities—often bringing heartache to themselves and to their parents.

Thus, the evolutionary "man as higher animal" assumption about human sexuality has conditioned teenage sexual education in the schools—and the consequences are everywhere. Educators who tell teenagers that sex is just part of growing up and that it can be a "loving and learning" experience outside of marriage don't understand that men and women are created by God "in His image" and are not the result of an amoral, animalistic, evolutionary process. God teaches that sex outside of marriage is wrong and that there will be consequences for such actions (1 Thessalonians 4:6).

Yet, of all the possible solutions to the sexual disaster of America, the most rational, most effective, and most powerful—abstinence—is frequently the most opposed and maligned. Why, for example, does the American Civil Liberties Union attempt to challenge abstinence-based programs on constitutional grounds when a personal decision to be abstinent is not *necessarily* related to religious beliefs at all?

Is it really unrealistic to expect young people to wait? Isn't it our *modern* attitudes and habits of sexuality that are unrealistic and dangerous? Isn't proof of this everywhere? Two generations ago abstinence was not considered "impossible," "unreasonable," or "dangerous." It was considered good and moral, and it was expected of young people.

And isn't it absurd to say that abstinence is unrealistic when non-abstinence can be fatal? In truth, isn't it those who have *encouraged* sexual permissiveness who are partly responsible for the suffering and deaths of others—and not those who have upheld abstinence?

A report on ABC News's "American Agenda" (April 1, 1992) was condescending to the abstinence-based national "Sex-Respect" program because it was supposedly based on "fear." Yet the same program described as "frightening" the great increase in AIDS and other STDs among teens. Eric Zorn, a columnist for the *Chicago Tribune*, in the September 20, 1992, issue also criticized abstinence promoting ads sponsored by Focus on the Family as being fear-based. Abstinence programs, however, are not based on fear, but they do warn about the serious consequences facing the sexually active. There are indeed things to fear today. To fail to warn teens about real dangers is not acting in their best interest.

To attack those who teach restraint as being foolish and unenlightened only worsens the problem. Further, in teaching that abstinence is only one of several approaches to containment, we help undermine the power of abstinence. Why? Because abstinence is less easily chosen when the more pleasant alternative of safe sex is held out as a "responsible" option.

What *safe sex* means is that activities God considers wrong and sinful—activities that frequently harm people regardless of what one thinks of them—are held out as safe and moral. But "safe anal intercourse," "safe fornication," and "safe adultery" are still anal intercourse, fornication, and adultery—and it is these activities that will continue to bring the consequences of the AIDS/STD plague upon us—physically, emotionally, socially, and economically.

What many sex educators and parents forget is that, in an age where the sex act can literally be lethal, premarital abstinence is the only guarantee of our children's safety. Teaching this is neither unrealistic nor moralistic and repressive. It is teaching a medical fact.

Does the problem lie at the door of adults for accepting the idea that their children can't control their sexual urges and then permitting sex educators to powerfully reinforce such a belief in the schools? If society treats kids like biological animals who have sexual instincts that cannot be controlled, should we be surprised at the outcome? But if society treats them as responsible young adults who are morally bound to control their sexual natures for their own welfare and that of society in general, then that is how they will model their behavior.

How do we know kids can say no? Because for most of human history the vast majority of teenagers have waited for sex until marriage. Even today one-third to one-half of all American teenagers are already saying no—they are not sexually involved. They could be if they wanted to, but they aren't. Teenagers adopt this behavior all over the world. In China the vast majority of teenagers—95 percent—remain chaste until marriage. The same is true in many other countries. Perhaps it is not true in America because we won't let it be true.

But there is no reason why things can't change. Shari and Tim are an example of an attitude and commitment to sane sexuality that can be found among thousands of teenagers across the country. In this case, both have been raised in strong Christian homes where biblical values are both taught and lived. Sexual issues have been discussed frankly, and the strong love that both teens feel from their parents has provided a foundation to resist temptations to sexual experimentation.

Both Tim and Shari had made personal commitments: first, to obeying God's will in their lives, and, second, to honoring their parents' instruction. Both were committed to being abstinent until marriage. And both succeeded. They are now happily married, beginning healthy families of their own.

MODERN CULTURAL ATTITUDES

Few will deny that how children are raised will play a crucial role in how they view sexual intercourse. But so will cultural attitudes. Whereas a good upbringing can inhibit peer pressure toward sexual experimentation, a poor home environment only tends to exacerbate the situation.

Social statistics reveal the wide range of sexual behavior among teenagers—in Sweden 90 percent have had sex before their twentieth birthday, but in Japan only 17 percent have had sex before age twenty (in America it's 65 percent).[6]

What makes the difference? As McDowell points out, certainly it is not that the young women in Japan have more character or power to say no than young women in Sweden or America. The issue isn't ability; teenagers are the same everywhere—they are all young adults with equal ability, morally speaking.[7] The real issue is the social and peer pressure teenagers face in American culture and the failure of adults to educate them in making the responsible choice of abstinence.

Isn't proof of this the fact that 30 years ago we had almost no problem with teenage abortion, widespread venereal disease, AIDS and sexual promiscuity? Teenagers who were pregnant were shunned and there was a general moral consensus giving virginity a positive social value. Moral standards were not only clearly defined; they were clearly spoken throughout the culture. Virginity was prized, not demeaned, and greater willingness existed from those in positions of power and influence to promote sexual chastity. But today, because of the "sexual freedom" groups, we have caved in to their agenda for society. Instead of acting wisely and with conviction, we have permitted them to dictate the rules of the game and offered no resistance.

In the 1950s to have a baby out of wedlock was a personal disgrace—the government would never have subsidized such a scandal. Today, the government does so, and the public demands it. The government also supports homosexuality, lesbianism, and the murder of children in the womb. Then it expects the public to fund the consequences of such activity—along with a failing Social Security system, AFDC (Aid to Families with Dependent Children), Medicaid, Savings and Loan scandals, bank failures, the FDIC, and so on.

To think that the government can now solve the sexual problems of the country by pouring billions of dollars into education—without fundamental attitude and behavior changes at all levels of society—represents a basic misunderstanding of human nature.

Why haven't billions of dollars spent on education and treatment programs significantly affected drug abuse in our country? Because we teach the wrong message. Illegal drugs are bad—but not bad enough to require sufficient penalties to curtail personal use. Millions of people enjoy drugs, and society is currently unwilling to take the necessary measures—stiff penalties for users—that would stop the epidemic.

Why haven't billions of dollars spent on "criminal justice," counseling, and legal services for offenders stopped crime in our country? Because we teach the wrong message. Crime is bad, but not so bad that we can't let murderers and other criminals out of jail on technicalities or reduce their sentences to just a few years because our jails are so overcrowded. So we let criminals out of jail (frequently after penalizing the victim) and then complain that crime is on the rise. What is the message to criminals? That chances are good they can get away with it. We give them this message and we then wonder why we have such a problem with repeat offenders.

In Italy the Mafia is so powerful that even though police have proof that some individuals have murdered as many as one-hundred-fifty to two-hundred people, yet they are powerless to stop them because of political corruption and liberal social policies. Given current policy in the United States, one only wonders how long it might be before America walks down a similar road.

We teach that religious values are good but simultaneously undermine their influence in society. Liberal social elements, such as the ACLU, work to prohibit religion and protect pornography and we wonder why we have a problem with child molestation, rape and other forms of violence against women.

The Clarence Thomas/Anita Hill debacle during Justice Thomas's confirmation hearings and the Navy's "Tailhook" scandal involving sexual harassment are illustrations of the problem. Many women's organizations around the country have, rightly, expressed concern over the subject of sexual harassment. Certainly, any nation that respects its women will not condone their mistreatment.

But we think that too many people are attacking symptoms rather than the problem. Perhaps consideration should also be given to garnering political power to confront the attitudes of sexual freedom in this country illustrated in such things as men's magazines and hard core pornography—or confronting the lack of concern for the sexual sanctity of marriage, seen in our adultery rates. Unfortunately, it appears that many of today's "liberated" men and women want to have their sexual freedom and so find it difficult to confront the root issues that give rise to problems like sexual harassment, rape, divorce and child abuse.

If there had continued a culture consensus—as was close to existing forty years ago—in accepting the biblical view of sexual morality, then as a nation, we would not have had to face either the root cause of our problems or its symptoms. As it stands, tremendous amounts of individual and political energy are being expended in attempting to deal with symptoms while root causes remain unaddressed. Until there is a return to promoting absolute moral standards in all segments of society, especially on the part of those who advocate moral change, we fear that such change will escape us.

Somehow we don't make a connection between children who are abducted, raped and murdered and the amoral sexual permissiveness in society. We accept tens of millions of abortions and then wonder why there are so few kids in school—complaining all the while that the government must subsidize schools to make up for declining enrollment. We officially reject religion-based morality, demand that discipline be removed from the school system and then complain about violence and absenteeism. And we wonder why there are thousands of illiterate children who never graduate from high school.

We say fiscal responsibility is good, but we encourage debt at every level of society—and then can't understand the bank failures, Savings and Loan scandals or a national debt that could produce a depression.

Now let's return to sex education. Is an "enjoy sex, but do it safely" mentality really educational? Or is it the problem? Can we tell kids that sex is entirely their own business and then expect them to behave responsibly at a young age?

Is it fair to educate our children in every aspect of sex—telling them in specific detail how to engage in the sexual act—and then expect them to be chaste? If our own children die of AIDS, whom should we blame? If we have ignored common sense, not to mention God, to whom do we turn for advice?

We cannot accept greed as a national standard and then wonder at the collapse of the stock market. We cannot accept politicians who reject absolute moral values and then wonder why the government is corrupt.

All these problems are symptoms of a two-faced morality that requires radical solution. Until the nation again adopts absolute moral values and widely promotes them, we will not see a change for the better.

In his November 6, 1992 interview on the Oprah Winfrey show, even Magic Johnson now says, "Abstinence is the key." In today's world, teaching abstinence is the only sane option. In the next several chapters we will reveal some of the consequences of adopting any other position.

ADDENDUM:
REASONS TO CONSIDER ABSTINENCE

- You will not get a sexually transmitted disease such asherpes, syphilis, clamydia, NGU, AIDS, etc.
- Your boyfriend, girlfriend or spouse will find it easier to trust you.
- God commands that sex is to be reserved for marriage.
- Premarital sex may make future courtship more problematic. It may also ruin what had previously been a good friendship, leaving pain, bitterness and mistrust. Abstinence permits freedom to develop a stronger friendship.
- Those who wait may find that the sexual relationship is perceived as being more special in marriage than those who do not wait.
- You will not have to deal with guilt, problems with self-esteem, or resentment on the part of another partner.
- Premarital sex will damage your relationship and walk with God.
- Ending a relationship after having premarital sex often leaves scars that are difficult to heal. It may also make it more difficult to break up with someone even if this is the best course of action.
- Premarital sex may break down communication within the relationship. Once begun, sex may be difficult to stop, and the desire for sex, rather than love, becomes predominant.
- You will not have to deal with the tremendous problem of unwanted pregnancy and abortion or the difficult task of raising children as a teenager or single parent.
- There is only one "first time."

- Studies have indicated that those who reserve sex for marriage often enjoy more satisfying sex and more stability in their marriage. Premarital sex may actually damage sexual fulfillment later in life.
- You will not have disobeyed God or be subject to His judgment.
- Those who have premarital sex have higher divorce rates.
- Premarital sex frequently makes it easier to justify extramarital sex. Your partner will be more confident that you will not engage in extramarital sex if you have not engaged in premarital sex.
- Premarital sex frequently harms your relationship with your parents.
- Premarital sex is a sin against your body (1 Corinthians 6:18). Waiting will bring God's blessing and self control and produce a feeling of personal self respect and dignity.
- Premarital sex may lead to further experimentation and even to various sexual addictions (e.g., pornography).
- Your sexual standards tend to influence those of your friends and others around you, whether for good or evil.
- Having premarital sex is a poor testimony for Christ.
- Waiting for your marriage partner is proof to that person of how much you love him or her.
- Those who have waited for sex until they are married have said they were not sorry they did so—yet countless numbers have regretted premarital sex.
- Premarital sex may induce a "performance syndrome," which unnecessarily complicates a relationship.
- Bad memories of broken relationships and friendships tend to stay with you and may damage your ability to trust others.
- Waiting brings true freedom.
- Premarital sex may make it difficult to make wise decisions regarding your relationship.
- Waiting until marriage will lead to good habit patterns in other areas of life.
- Premarital sex may have negative effects on your children, such as your inability to be a good role model in encouraging your own sons' and daughters' chastity.
- The consequences of premarital sex may hurt your reputation.
- The consequences of premarital sex are extremely harmful to society as a whole.

Sexually Transmitted Diseases: Fifty-seven and Counting*

Their Extraordinary Cost to Society

The damaging effects of STD's can be mild, but extremely aggravating, or they can be severe and permanent—as in death. . . . It seems that every few years human beings are assaulted (literally, battered) with new sexually transmitted diseases. Each succeeding disease seems worse than the last. . . . Most STD germs are very fragile . . . outside the body. . . . Inside the body, however, STD germs are extremely potent and can cause tremendous damage.

Joe McIlhaney, M.D.
Sexuality and Sexually Transmitted Diseases

The Guiness Book of World Records does not yet have a category for the individual with the most sexually transmitted diseases, but "Hud" might as well submit a report. Hud claims that he has had sexual encounters with more than eight thousand different men and women. In a period of ten years he has contracted herpes, chlamydia, syphilis, gonorrhea, chancroid, a multidrug resistant form of tuberculosis, scabies, genital warts, and thirteen other diseases related to his sexual practices. In fact, he has contracted these diseases a total of sixty-seven times. Surprisingly, he has not yet contracted AIDS.

It might not matter. Doctors have told him that his life span may have been reduced by as much as fifteen years—which means he may

---

* Documentation for the following can be found in journals such as *Sexually Transmitted Diseases Bulletin* (1980–), publications of the yearly World Congress on Sexually Transmitted Diseases (1985–), and related periodicals listed by medical indexes; Joe S. McIlhaney, Jr., M.D., *Sexuality and Sexually Transmitted Diseases* (1990); K. K. Holmes et al., eds., *Sexually Transmitted Diseases* (1990); Josh McDowell, *Research Almanac and Statistical Digest* (1991), and the Centers for Disease Control *Morbidity and Mortality Weekly Report*.

not have long to live. Although Hud is clearly the exception, it is becoming more and more common for people to encounter multiple sexually transmitted diseases in their lifetimes.

THE STD EXPLOSION

Apart from the common cold and flu, sexually transmitted diseases are now the most common diseases in America.[1] In fact, "These diseases are spreading like a firestorm in our country."[2]

But worldwide the picture is just as dismal. The World Health Organization estimates there are 250 million (one-quarter *billion*) cases of STDs each year.[3] Unfortunately, it could be that the battle to control these diseases is lost.

In that it was largely persons having liberal attitudes on sex who have helped produce the current epidemics—not those who have advocated abstinence—it is somewhat unrealistic for these persons to now attack the position of abstinence—our only safe recourse—as "unrealistic and harmful." In this chapter we will document why it is the liberal, permissive view of sex that is "unrealistic and harmful." In fact, the current epidemics will not cease until parents, teenagers and the rest of society understand fully the devastating consequences of sexual promiscuity—and act accordingly. For example: "STDs have touched the lives of everyone from innocent spouses to a celibate nun, resulting in birth defects, cancer, sterility, and death among men, women, and even children, who never knew they had a disease. And the problem is expected to escalate to incredible proportions."[4]

Leanne and Henry had been dating for about a year. They soon entered into an uncertain stage of their relationship and both decided to begin dating other people. Unfortunately, this led to sexual experimentation with others, hoping to discover if they really were "right" for each other.

Both affairs turned out poorly, and soon Leanne and Henry were back together. Leanne never realized she contracted both herpes and pelvic inflammatory disease (PID) from what she thought was one of the nicest, kindest men she had ever met. Henry never realized that he had contracted syphilis.

Within a month of recontinuing sexual intercourse, they had each passed their diseases to the other. Leanne was furious with Henry and vice versa; their mutual trust had been destroyed. Needless to say, the relationship didn't survive.

In recent years, the most noted STDs have been AIDS and herpes. But many other STDs constitute as serious a problem. For example, in the same ten years since AIDS first appeared, *other* STDs are estimated to have caused up to ninety fatalities as well as fetal and infant deaths in the *millions*.[5] Gonorrhea, syphilis and chancroid are now "increasing at epidemic rates among urban minority populations in the U.S."[6] Further, each year more babies are born with birth defects caused by STDs than all the children afflicted by polio during the entire ten-year epidemic of the 1950s.[7]

Most people have no idea of the collective damage caused by sexually transmitted diseases. Since the "sexual revolution" began thirty years ago, the result has been nothing short of incredible.

In twenty years hardly anyone will risk sex outside of certain knowledge of an uninfected, monogamous partner. Until that time, among literally tens of millions of people the message will either go unheard or unheeded, making the present years the most dangerous of all for risk of infection.

As far back as April 1981, *The Harvard Medical School Health Letter* noted the existence of 20 different STDs and the greater concern emerging among professionals was not the immediate symptoms of the STDs, but "their role in causing birth defects, infertility, and long term disability."[8]

Three years later *American Health* magazine reported on twenty-eight different STDs. It noted that this was the biggest explosion of "social diseases" since Columbus. It said that beyond the dread of AIDS "a savage variety of lesser known ailments" now infect Americans.[9] Further, "in romantic moments each year, ten to fifteen million citizens now enroll each other as victims of sexually transmitted diseases."[10] And, "at last count, twenty-eight different viruses, bacteria, fungi and parasites get exchanged with awesome frequency."[11]

On July 14, 1988, *The New York Times* reported fifty-one STDs and their numbers are increasing. In other words, thirty years ago there were only a few sexually transmitted diseases—the principal concerns were syphilis and gonorrhea. In 1992 we are approaching sixty, and apparently a new one is discovered every nine months.[12]

What's worse, many of these diseases are asymptomatic or mimic other illnesses and, therefore, are difficult to diagnose. For the majority of the most common STDs "there is on the average a 40 to 60 percent chance that you will have *no discernible symptoms* or will mistake them for something else."[13] Thus, women who do have the characteristic signs of an STD are easily misdiagnosed. For example, pelvic pain, painful intercourse, fever, abnormal discharges or bleeding from the vagina, nausea and vomiting, pain with urinating or defecating—may receive a false diagnosis of bladder infection (cystitis) because the symptoms are so similar. Without proper tests for various STDs, the condition will progress unobstructed, frequently to the point where the damage is done and it is too late to help. (The best way to diagnose PID, for example, is a small operation called laparoscopy, which allows the physician to examine the tubes for inflammation and get specimens for culture). Unfortunately, as with AIDS, many people resist testing for fear of the consequences. No one likes being diagnosed as having a sexually transmitted disease. But the consequences of not being diagnosed are far worse.

THE CONSEQUENCES OF STDS

Ten to twenty million American women are now sterile because of sexual infections from promiscuity; the figures may go as high as one-fourth of all women of childbearing age.[14] That is a terrible price to pay for a few moments of pleasure.

Regardless, apparently twelve to fifteen million new cases of sexually transmitted diseases occur each year. "Statistics show that the incidence of nearly every STD is on the rise."[15] Somewhere between thirty-five and forty thousand Americans acquire an STD every *day* of the year.[16] This means that at least 25 percent—or one in every four—of Americans between the ages of fifteen and fifty-five will eventually acquire a sexually transmitted disease.[17] And the figures may run higher.

Further, STDs are frequently synergistic, having a combined effect surpassing that of their individual infections. For example, concurrent infections with gonorrhea and chlamydia greatly increase the risk of PID and infertility when compared to these infections alone. Further, many STDs, such as syphilis and herpes, actually increase a person's risk for AIDS infection.

Herb was not particularly sexually active. He had been with only a few women before he met his "true love." Sharon was much more sexually active than Herb and in the past year had contracted both herpes and chancroid. But Herb loved her and wanted to marry her.

Unfortunately, what Sharon couldn't know (later confirmed by doctors) was that her forthcoming diagnosis of HIV infection was probably attributable to her earlier exposure to other STDs. Tragically, after her diagnosis, she discovered she had passed on the HIV virus to Herb. As of this writing, Herb is dead. Sharon is in the hospital and weighs less than sixty pounds. She is not expected to survive the month.

Scientific American reported the following in 1991: "This increase [in chancroid rates] could have profound public health consequences because chancroid may facilitate HIV transmission. Worse still, the bacterium that causes chancroid has developed resistance to many antimicrobial drugs. In persons who have been exposed to HIV, chancroid often fails to respond to some therapies that are otherwise highly effective. Thus, HIV infection may help the spread of a bacterial STD that in turn helps to spread HIV."[18]

> The evidence that other STD's increase the sexual transmission of HIV can be summarized as follows. The STD's that cause genital ulcer disease—chancroid, syphilis and genital herpes—have been associated with an increased risk of acquiring HIV infection in heterosexual men and women in Africa. Syphilis and herpes have also been associated with HIV infection in heterosexual men and women and in homosexual men in the U.S. In African women the risk of heterosexual acquisition of HIV has been elevated in those with gonorrhea or chlamydial infection of the cervix or those with a form of vaginal discharge caused by *Trichomonas,* a common parasite.
>
> Conversely, HIV infection leads to altered manifestations of other STD and thereby probably promotes their spread. Genital and anorectal herpes ulcers normally heal within one to three weeks, but they may persist for months as highly infectious ulcers in persons with HIV infection. As previously noted, HIV infection also raises the risk of treatment failure for chancroid ulcers. There is anecdotal evidence for the failure of syphilis treatments and for altered manifestations of syphilis and gonorrhea in HIV-positive persons. We can, therefore, postulate that HIV and other STD may promote one another's spread.[19]

Then there are other possible synergisms. *Science News* reported that those women infected with certain types of HPV (human papilloma virus) who also smoke tobacco may be at greater risk for cervical cancer.[20]

What's worse, "teenagers have more STD's than any other group in the United States."[21] Each year some three million of them acquire STDs and 25 percent of all the sexually active will get one before graduating.[22] Again, every year one in seven teenagers contracts an STD, making STDs epidemic among teens as well: [23] "While the STD rate is severe for the population as a whole, the rate in the 16 to 20 year-old age group is three times that of the general population. For example, Chlamydia has become the most commonly diagnosed STD, and among sexually active teens, its prevalence may be as high as 30 percent. Its incidence in teens can be called epidemic. Other STDs are also increasing among teens. Cervical cancer, now classified as an STD, is a problem especially among young teens. . . . The prevalence among sexually active teens is estimated to be 11–22 percent."[24] Doesn't this suggest that millions of our children are suffering because, as a nation, we lacked the common sense to teach them abstinence?[25]

Teenagers, like many of their parents, frequently ignore the consequences of their sexual activity. Consider the letter to "Dear Abby" as reported in the *Los Angeles Times* for October 16, 1979. A sixteen-year-old girl had thanked Abby for a column on STDs. She wished she had seen something like this a few years earlier. She explained that at sixteen, she had just undergone a "very painful and serious" hysterectomy as a result of contracting gonorrhea. This teenager noted that she was not promiscuous and had never slept around. She had only one boyfriend. Now she had a seven inch scar on her stomach. She confessed that the worst part was knowing that she would never be able to have children. She concluded that most kids do not understand how serious STDs are, and signed her letter, "Paid a High Price."

Unfortunately, viral STDs such as HPV, AIDS, herpes, and hepatitis are with a person for life and have no cure. Some *fifty million* Americans now carry one or more of these viruses in their bodies and will have to live with them permanently.[26]

Nor are married men and women safe if their partners are sexually unfaithful. Josh McDowell, who has spoken to more than ten million people on the subject of human sexuality, reports:

> Last fall . . . 24 women spoke to me who were each carrying three to six sexually transmitted diseases they had contracted from their husbands. Many of the diseases were incurable and/or cancer producing. Several of the women said that their doctors strongly admonished them to be tested for cancer every six months—for the rest of their lives. When their husbands played around sexually, some before marriage and some after, they weren't just participating in innocent, private affairs. Their so-called private acts will affect their wives and children for as long as any of them live.[27]

Even while a person is without symptoms and the STD is dormant, it can be transmitted to anyone else that person has sex with. Edward Wiesmeier, director of the UCLA Student Health Center warns, "One chance encounter can infect a person with as many as five different diseases."[28]

FACTS ABOUT THE MOST COMMON STDS

AIDS:

- Twenty percent of all people with AIDS are in their twenties, many of them infected during their teenage years.
- Infants born to infected mothers have a one-in-ten to one-in-three chance of testing positive for HIV depending on the stage of HIV infection (early or late).[29] This means that eventually millions of children will be infected. Without a cure, all will die.
- UNICEF estimates that by 1999 almost thirty million children will be orphaned by AIDS.[30]
- Because AIDS destroys the immune system, making the body susceptible to a large number of damaging or fatal illnesses it could otherwise ward off, the means by which most people die of AIDS are more painful, disfiguring, and traumatic than many other illnesses. By the time a person has died from AIDS he may have had various types of pneumonia, debilitating fungus infections, tuberculosis, syphilis, severe forms of common infections, various cancers, severe brain damage involving dementia, seizures, and so on.[31]
- In the brief few years AIDS has existed, it has become the leading cause of death for single American men between the ages of fifteen and fifty. Among teens the number of cases is doubling every fourteen months, and more teenagers now get AIDS heterosexually than adults.
- Before the epidemic is over, a few authorities have estimated that, without a cure, between 500 million and two billion could die.

Thankfully, current research seems increasingly promising—and we just may find a vaccine or cure. Unfortunately it appears that it will not be before at least fifty million people are dead.

Herpes:

- By 1988, forty million Americans were infected with herpes—more than one-half million are newly infected each year.[32] Characteristically, an individual may not have physical symptoms.[33]

- Although estimates vary, it would seem that between one-third and one-half of all adults carry the genital herpes virus in their blood stream. A JAMA study as far back as 1986 indicated that "the average adult male in the United States has almost a 50 percent chance of having already been infected with the virus."[34] Further, according to Masters and Johnson, "The risk of developing genital herpes in a woman exposed to an infected man is estimated to be 80 to 90 percent."[35]
- Again, one-third to more than one-half of initial herpes infections are symptomless or go unnoticed. Such persons who continue to have sex continue to infect others. "Remember, that 75 percent of herpes-infected individuals have never had an outbreak of herpes (and, therefore, may be unaware of its existence), but can pass it on nonetheless."[36]
- There is even a new strain of herpes that is entirely asymptomatic. (Like the AIDS virus, other STDs are also mutating into different forms.) This new strain is impossible to detect until the woman has a child born with a birth defect.[37]
- In common with other viruses, herpes cannot successfully be treated with antibiotics although some antiviral agents may suppress the infection and its characteristic recurrences.
- Herpes can spread to others even when condoms are used.
- Babies vaginally delivered to mothers with a primary outbreak of infection have a high chance of contracting the disease (60 percent or more of these may die and most others will suffer brain damage). This requires delivery by C-section if the mother is known to have an active infection or shedding herpes viruses.
- Rarely, herpes infects the brain causing severe brain damage or death. It has also been associated with cancer of the cervix.[38]
- As with AIDS, just one sexual experience with a symptom-free but infected person may lead to years of intermittent suffering.

NGU/MCP:

- Nongonococcal urethritis (NGU) and mucopurulent cervicitis (MPC) refer to a variety of diseases that affect men and women respectively. NGU is any infection of the urethra not due to gonorrhea and is also known as NSU or nonspecific urethritis. Frequently, NGU and MPC are lumped together under NGU.
- About half of all cases in men are caused by the organism chlamydia trachomatis, which is also responsible for about one-quarter million cases of acute epididymitis each year.[39] (Epididymitis infects the ducts carrying the sperm from the testicles, causing sterility.)
- In women, chlamydia trachomatis accounts for an estimated one-quarter to one-half million cases of PID per year[40] (see below).
- *Reader's Digest* reported in November 1979 that NGU (which it described as "an insidious disease") had become the most common venereal infection in the U.S., England, and other developed countries. Victims of NGU outnumbered those of gonorrhea by two to one—four to nine million cases each year. Symptoms of NGU in men are similar to those of gonorrhea but deceptively milder. Infected women frequently have no symptoms. NGU can cause Reiter's syndrome, an especially painful form of arthritis. In addition, 75 percent of epididymitis cases involving men

under thirty-five were traceable to NGU.
- NGU also sterilizes women by infecting and closing the fallopian tubes.
- From 1965 to 1980 tubal pregnancies tripled in America, partly the result of epidemics of gonorrhea and NGU. Unfortunately, pregnancy itself makes women more susceptible to NGU—the disease can infect the womb after delivery. But it is even more of a menace to babies. *Reader's Digest* described the effects of NGU upon "tortured babies," noting, "Venereal diseases have been a medical wasteland in this country." Today, NGU/MPC continues to infect men and women at epidemic rates.[41]

PID:

- Pelvic inflammatory disease also strikes about one million American women each year and is caused by a variety of bacteria or other organisms such as chlamydia trachomatis. It is a major cause of infertility and ectopic pregnancy. In 1991 we spent four billion dollars treating this disease and will spend at least ten to twenty billion more by the year 2000. According to STD specialist Judith Wasserheit of the National Institute of Allergy and Infectious Diseases, by 2000 A.D. about 50 percent of all women will have contracted PID.[42]
- Although PID is a "silent epidemic" usually infecting women, it can also affect men—without symptoms—and, rarely, it can even be fatal. In some cases, a severe infection is produced. Without surgery, the patient may die within a matter of hours, but the surgery itself may involve removing the reproductive organs, leaving the woman unable to bear children.
- Even when PID involves very mild infections, it may still lead to complete blockage of the fallopian tubes and infertility from scarring. Many women never suspect something is wrong until they attempt to get pregnant and discover they cannot.
- PID may cause miscarriages and premature labor, stillbirths and postpartum infection. In newborn children it may cause eye infections and pneumonia.[43] Chlamydia trachomatis, which also causes PID, is more common than gonorrhea and syphilis combined, presenting about four million new cases every year.[44] Each year combined costs of chlamydia are $1.5 to $2.5 billion.[45] With chlamydial infection, up to half of all women have no symptoms when they are infected.[46]
- As is true for many other STDs, infected women may not discover the results of their sexual activity until they attempt to get pregnant or discover they have infected their babies:[47]

  > Maternal chlamydial infections during pregnancy are commonly passed to the newborn during childbirth, presumably from the infant coming in contact with infected secretions in the birth canal. Up to 50 percent of infants born to infected mothers develop conjunctivitis (a type of eye infection), and 3 to 18 percent develop chlamydial pneumonia (a lung infection) before they are four months old. While chlamydial pneumonia is not usually serious, chlamydial conjunctivitis can sometimes cause chronic eye disease. . . . A number of studies also link chlamydial infections with various complications of pregnancy, such as premature rupture of the fetal membranes, premature delivery, and postpartum endometritis.[48]

- *Scientific American* noted that "silent but destructive disease is the hall-mark of chronic chlamydial infection."[49] In fact, permitting an infection to "burn in your body without treatment even a few days too long" greatly increases chances of sterility.[50]
- Women who develop PID as a result of chlamydia, gonorrhea, or another bacterial infection have a 10 to 15 percent chance of becoming permanently infertile on their first infection, a 30 to 35 percent chance on their second, and a 60 to 75 percent chance on their third. Each year twenty thousand women become infertile from chlamydia infections alone.[51]
- PID may lead to ectopic pregnancy, which has experienced a dramatic rise in the past decade; 50 percent of those who have ectopic pregnancies become infertile.
- *Science News* reported that because of STDs ectopic pregnancy "now ranks as the leading cause of pregnancy-related death among women in the first trimester."[52]
- Condoms do not prevent the spread of chlamydia.

CMV:

- Like many other STDs, cytomegalovirus frequently produces no symptoms, but may cause illnesses similar to flu or mononucleosis.
- An estimated forty to eighty thousand babies were born in 1982 with congenital CMV infections; 10 to 20 percent have significant or permanent handicaps, including small or large headedness, seizures, psychomotor retardation, and hearing and learning problems. Other babies will die before birth, be born prematurely, or have fatal problems of the liver and spleen. It may also cause pneumonia and other respiratory problems in babies.

Hepatitis B:

- Hepatitis B is another common viral STD, presenting 300,000 new cases per year in the U.S., with some 200 million carriers throughout the world.[53]
- Approximately 60 percent of all homosexual men have had hepatitis, with 85 percent becoming infected by age forty.[54]
- Mild cases of hepatitis result in flu-like symptoms or no symptoms at all; severe cases may result in fatal liver damage or cancer.[55]
- Hepatitis can be transmitted to an unborn child resulting in its death, a stillbirth, premature delivery, or ongoing infection through childhood. Some research indicates that 90 percent of babies born to mothers who are chronic hepatitis B virus carriers will be infected at the time of birth; of these, 90 percent will become chronic hepatitis B carriers themselves.[56]

Venereal Warts and HPV:

- Human papilloma virus is a common STD linked to cervical and other cancers.
- The *Los Angeles Times* of October 8, 1983, reported that every year cervical cancer is expected to strike sixteen thousand American women, causing seven thousand deaths. It noted that a new STD was spreading to more people than both herpes and AIDS combined. In 1981 nearly one million people were treated for HPV.

- But on January 23, 1991, *USA Today* reported that HPV has now "reached epidemic proportions in sexually active youth." Indeed, almost *half* of all sexually active college women may now be infected.[57] Every year one or two million new cases of venereal warts are reported in the U.S. and, currently, up to *twenty-four million* people are believed to be infected with HPV.[58]
- This disease starts as little more than a nuisance—genital warts—but can result in cervical cancer in women and other genital cancers in both sexes.[59] Once exposed, a person may be predisposed to cancer by one of several mechanisms—for example, the herpes virus interacting with the papilloma virus, or excessive exposure to sunlight.
- Sometimes genital warts go away. Usually, they spread and become uncomfortable or disfiguring. Treatments include surgery, burning, freezing, or chemical removal. As with herpes, women with genital warts should have frequent pap smears because of the cancer link. Thus, HPV is thought to be a contributing factor in "cervical, vaginal, and vulvar intraepithelial neoplasia and carcinoma."[60] About eight thousand women die each year from HPV associated cancers.[61]
- Sixty percent of the sexual partners of patients with venereal warts have the infection themselves.
- Other sexually transmitted diseases such as syphilis, gonorrhea, and trichomoniasis are frequently found along with venereal warts.
- Venereal warts may interfere with the delivery of a child.
- Women who have venereal warts, secondary to the human papilloma virus infection, are much more likely to have cervical cancer than women without the warts.
- Certain types of human papilloma virus are found in more than 90 percent of cervical cancers studied. *Family Practice News* of August 1–14, 1984, reported that "an epidemic of cervical cancer among women is likely to occur if liberal sexual lifestyles continue."[62] (See note 62 for more.)

Syphilis:

- In the last ten years there has been a dramatic increase in the number of syphilis cases, which has five main stages.[63]
- Syphilis is a potentially severe STD that may produce heart, brain, and spinal cord damage leading to a variety of debilitating conditions, including death. Syphilis of the brain can mimic almost any psychiatric disorder and some data link syphilitic infection with increased rates of AIDS infection.
- "[In] . . . *Benign Diseases of the Vulva and Vagina*, Drs. Herman L. Gardner and Raymond Kaufman write: . . . 'According to estimates, approximately half of the patients with syphilis are either unaware of its presence, or consider the lesions inconsequential until the disease is past its early stages.' . . .

  "When syphilis reaches the late stage, it can produce devastating medical problems in almost any part of the body. Some of the more common effects are aneurysms of the cardiovascular system, deterioration of the central nervous system, involvement of bones, and damage to peripheral nerves. . . . During the latent stage, the syphilis spirochetes do tremendous damage throughout the body. Large abscesses are formed and entire organs can be destroyed. Once well into the latent stage, a patient may sustain irreversible damage to the bones, liver cells, heart valves, blood vessels, and central nervous system."[64]

- Congenital infections have increased fourfold from 1985 to 1987 and have continued to rise. About 25 percent of infected children die before birth, another 25 percent die shortly after birth and many others develop various complications.[65]

  There is one major threat that occurs during all stages of syphilis—damage to the unborn child of a syphilitic mother. Babies can develop syphilis while still in their mother's womb, and congenital syphilis is a disaster. Such pregnancies often end in spontaneous miscarriages or stillbirths. Other infected babies die soon after birth. Those that live are often born with such abnormalities as nose obstruction, flattening of the bridge of the nose, fractures of the bones, enlarged liver and spleen, and eye or ear damage. *Population Reports* (July 1983) quotes a study showing that of 220 pregnancies in women with untreated primary or secondary syphilis, 38 percent ended in spontaneous miscarriages, still-births, or neonatal death; and 41 percent resulted in the birth of a syphilitic infant.[66]

Gonorrhea:

- Gonorrhea has become "the most common reportable disease in school-age children, surpassing chicken pox, measles, mumps and rubella combined."[67] The highest rate of gonorrhea infection of any age group is the fifteen- to nineteen-year-old category. Gonorrhea is also the principal cause of arthritis in young adults. One to two million new cases are reported each year.
- In women, gonorrhea may cause PID leading to infertility or ectopic pregnancy.
- Sixty percent of women and 20 percent of men with a gonorrhea infection have no symptoms, making treatment and spread of the disease difficult to control.
- As is true for several other STDs, gonorrhea is increasingly resistant to penicillin even while it continues to develop resistant strains.

Other STDs:

- Trichomoniasis affects about 20 percent of all women who are sexually active with multiple partners during the reproductive years. There are an estimated three million or more new cases in the U.S. every year[68] with one study reporting eight million.[69] This disease may also increase risk of infertility in women.
- Ureaplasma (T-mycolplasma) is a temporary cause of infertility in women and may play a role in miscarriages; in men it may lead to urethritis, conjunctivitis, and arthritis.
- There is also gardnerella vaginalis or hemophilus, chanchroid, LVG (lymphgramuloma venereum), GI (granuloma inguinale), molluscum contagiosum, Epstein-Barr, virus, and three dozen more STDs too numerous to list. "Chanchroid, GI, and LGV are highly dangerous and destructive diseases causing the loss of vital tissues in the reproductive organs, gross

> enlargement of the sex organs, stricture of the intestines and rectum, obstruction of the anus, even death."[70]

Unfortunately, with the large number of STDs that have emerged in the last thirty years, research is consistently behind in determining the exact consequences of most of them. Although drugs and other treatments have proved successful for many, we still don't know the long-term consequences for others.

But additional research is not the solution. STDs may never be controlled medically because they are growing at too fast a rate. They may also mutate. Again, the only solution is a radical change in sexual attitudes and behavior.

To risk infertility, life-long pain, cancer and other diseases—or even death—is absurd. To teach our own children and the rest of society that safe sex is the solution seems almost criminal.

In spite of the repeated degrading of Christian values in this country, the simple fact is that abiding by those values would have prevented the entire STD epidemic. It is surprising that nearly 2,000 years ago God warned through the apostle Paul: "Flee from sexual immorality. All other sins a man commits are outside his body, but he who sins sexually sins against his own body" (1 Corinthians 6:18).

The words of Dr. McIlhaney appropriately conclude this chapter: "If sex is avoided until marriage and then engaged in only in marriage, all these sexually transmitted diseases would be of no importance at all because they could not enter into a closed circle relationship between husband and wife. Such an approach is not only not naive, it is also not moralizing, but it is now necessary." [71]

6

AIDS

Will It Become a Worldwide Plague of Unprecedented Proportions?

AIDS is the most significant threat to the human race in the modern era.

Joseph Feldschuch, M.D.

We are indeed at war with a virus quite capable of destroying our civilization.

David Pence, M.D.

According to a comprehensive study just released by Harvard University, by the end of the decade between 30 and 110 million adults, plus 10 million children worldwide, will have HIV. The study concluded that the world is reacting far too slowly to the epidemic.[1]

James and Sandra were the quintessentially happily married couple. They had everything going for them, including a beautiful, precocious child. The last thing they expected to encounter was a virus that could destroy their lives. But in 1985 their son, Jason, required a blood transfusion after hemorrhaging during a routine tonsillectomy. Three years later they discovered he was infected with HIV. They were shattered.

The next several years were spent in agony, watching their beloved child die. Today they still cannot fathom how the local blood banks and federal government could have permitted the blood supply to be contaminated. They no longer trust civil government and, in fact, blame it for their child's death. They believe that, if the government had spent less time being concerned about the "civil rights" of alternate sexual lifestyles and more time instituting standard public health measures, Jason would be alive. "No one knows the bitterness in my heart," says Sandra. "I will never forget, and I will never forgive."

One AIDS patient describes his losing battle with HIV: "The fear. The pain. Living with AIDS is horrible. You never know how you're going to feel at any time, on any day. You wait to die while the terror increases."

AIDS is undoubtedly the most lethal STD. Thankfully, new research shows a little promise, at least concerning a vaccine (see below).

THE AIDS INFECTION

There are currently six stages in the development of AIDS,[2] although it must be remembered that the vast majority of those who are HIV positive will contract the disease and die. For reasons that are not entirely clear, a person is diagnosed as having AIDS only at the end stages of the illness. More appropriate revisions in classification may now be underway, but at the time of writing the following stages are accepted:

Stage 1– The Initial Infection

The virus causing AIDS enters the blood and quickly penetrates mostly the white "T4" cells in the body, the key coordinators of the immune system— although brain, and certain other, cells may also be affected. It programs these cells in such a manner that "there is often no trace of the virus [left] at all."[3] In other words, the virus has a "stealth" capacity, making it invisible not only to medical tests but to the body's own immune system. In part, that is what permits the virus to replicate and gain a stronghold in the body. This situation usually lasts for six weeks or more (in some people up to fourteen months, perhaps longer), and during this period the person is free of symptoms, and all current tests are negative.[4]

Stage 2 – Flu-like Illnesses

Once infected cells begin to die, many people develop flu-like symptoms. The symptoms may vary from moderate to severe. It is at this point that the body begins to produce antibodies that may be picked up by testing.

Stage 3 – The "Body Positive" Stage

The person nearly always has a positive test but feels completely well. The virus may then completely disappear from the blood.

Stage 4 – The PGL Stage

Here the immune system begins to break down. Glands in the armpits and neck may swell and remain swollen for three months or more without explanation. This is known as persistent generalized lymphadenopathy (PGL).

Stage 5 – The ARC Stage

As the disease progresses, individuals develop other conditions related to AIDS. Boils or warts may spread over the body. People may experience extreme tiredness, high temperatures, drenching night sweats, lose more than 10 percent of their body weight, and have diarrhea for more than a month. This is called AIDS related complex or AIDS related condition (ARC).

Stage 6 – Full-Blown AIDS

This is the stage at which opportunistic infections become a nightmare for the one infected—as well as for his doctors. It is a constant battle to determine what the infection is and how to best treat it. Further, it is now known that the AIDS virus itself does directly attack the body, e.g., the brain. It does not merely suppress the immune system, thereby opening the body to a variety of general infections.

It is now easy to see that many people who could have died of AIDS in years past may have been diagnosed as having died from some other condition. The agents that eventually kill the individual, because his immune system is suppressed, may be hiding deep in the lungs, the brain, spinal cord, gall bladder, bowel, heart—anywhere. One of the most common infections is of the lung,[5] but "HIV itself seems to attack, damage and destroy brain cells of the majority of people with AIDS who survive long enough."[6] Further, "almost all people with AIDS have stomach problems from strange infections and cancers caused by AIDS and HIV attacking the gut directly. . . . AIDS can also seriously affect sight by allowing an infection of the back of the eye (retinitis)."[7]

THE AIDS VIRUS

The virus that causes AIDS is called HIV (Human Immunodeficiancy Virus). It is incredibly small. While thousands of bacteria can fit inside a single cell in the human body, *virus* particles are so diminutive that literally *hundreds* of thousands of them can fit inside a single *bacterium*. All viruses do not need food to survive, nor do they breathe. They cannot grow, divide, do not live, and never die, although they *can* be killed. "All our technology has failed to produce a single drug that attacks and destroys a virus directly."[8] In other words, the only weapons against viruses are natural ones—human antibodies produced by our immune systems to destroy them.

The trouble with antibodies is that the body takes three days to produce the right antibody for the right virus. During this critical three-day period, the body is totally unprotected. Yet only an hour or two after viruses have entered the bloodstream, they have completely disappeared. You can hunt through the entire body, cell by cell, with the best electron firing microscope and find nothing.

Why? Because every virus particle has disintegrated. Each one has burst like a child's soap bubble when it touches the ground.

The virus bag has disintegrated and vanished. What about the contents?

They too have disappeared without trace, but the cell it touched has received the kiss of death.[9]

How does the HIV destroy the cell? Dr. Patrick Dixon explains: "When HIV touches a cell and the bubble bursts, the genetic code is injected suddenly into the cell. Within minutes the code is being read by the cell and the message is being carried into the cell's brain, or nucleus. The message is then added permanently to that cell's 'book of life.' The process took only a few minutes and is complete. The cell looks normal in every way but is now doomed. It may continue to look normal for several years. During this time the white cell continues to travel in the blood looking for invaders while blissfully unaware of the invader within. If the attacked cell divides, the two daughter cells also carry perfect copies of the hidden message."[10]

What this means is that every cell infected with HIV becomes a kind of "biological time bomb" traveling throughout the bloodstream. Soon, literally millions of them are just waiting to explode. The AIDS virus has ignored most other cells and honed in on the master coordinator of the immune system, the helper T-cell. Once on the surface of the cell it finds a receptor into which one of its proteins fits perfectly, as a key into a lock. The virus penetrates the cell membrane and an incredible transformation begins. The virus starts to reproduce itself. After penetrating the cell nucleus, it inserts itself into a chromosome and takes over part of the cellular machinery, actually commanding it to produce more AIDS viruses.[11] Remarkably, the virus has actually overridden the normal DNA message (to produce antibodies) and instead produces more HIV.

In other words, once infected with AIDS, the body becomes its own worst enemy. Thus, "infected white cells become factories for more virus, instead of factories to help the body make antibodies."[12] Eventually sufficient numbers of the AIDS virus are produced so that the cell swells and dies, releasing millions of HIV particles in the process. These in turn attack other cells including more helper T-cells: "You can see special electron microscope photographs of hundreds of these viruses appearing as little bulges as they poke out from the cell. Eventually they emerge as little round balls, and the cell dies. Millions of virus particles are released into the bloodstream, each one floating in the blood until it touches another T4 white cell, bursts, injects its message, reprograms the cell, and the process continues."[13]

Even with modern technology we still find it nearly impossible to detect an infected cell. Until they are actually dying, they appear identical to a healthy cell. But the problem with HIV is not that the body cannot produce antibodies against the virus. It produces antibodies that enable us to diagnose someone as being infected. But "the sinister thing is that the virus is *immune* to antibodies. No antibodies have yet been found in a human being that are effective against HIV. That is why a vaccine will be so difficult to find. It is easy to produce antibodies against the virus, but we don't know how to produce one that will prevent infection because we have no natural models from which to work."[14]

Unfortunately, it seems that in AIDS research, early claims to success are often tempered down the road. Current approaches are operating on several fronts. For example, one program is attempting to develop a protein that attaches to the virus and inhibits its reproduction; but no one can say how successful this will prove. The partial vaccine GP–160 was first thought to be a breakthrough, but recent news reports have tempered enthusiasm. Nevertheless, the research behind it illustrates how researchers are proceeding.

Dr. Robert Redfield is with the Division of Retrovirology, Walter Reed Army Institute of Research. By using a specially cultured outer-sheath of HIV as a "vaccine" he found a way to undermine the virus "stealth" capacity (by which it is indetectible to antibodies), thus permitting the body and its immune system greater knowledge of HIV infection. This gives the body a better chance to fight the virus. In an interview conducted for The John Ankerberg Show, Redfield explained his discovery:

> We actually took the gene that makes the outside of the AIDS virus—proteins—there's two of them—and we put that gene into a factory cell in the test tube, and that factory cell now made that protein—actually, it made the parent protein. These two outside proteins—when they're made naturally and then get split—they make two separate proteins. What we did was

we made the parent protein. In other words, *both* of the proteins that make up the outside envelope of the HIV virus. And then you purify that protein so you don't have virus—it's not infectious, it's just the outside protein. It doesn't cause HIV infection. And we took that, and we actually vaccinated patients that were already infected. What we showed was although these patients make the same protein in their body and don't see it, when we vaccinate them, we teach them to see it. We are actually *teaching* the body to do what it would like to do to make HIV not chronic. And I think that's the net outcome. Down the line we are going to make HIV nonchronic. But it's going to be stepwise.

Hopefully over the future we'll learn—and I think we've made a lot of progress so far in potentially modifying the disease, but by no means do I want people to believe that I think that I've stopped the disease. We've *modified* it so we've gained a little. I use a baseball analogy. I think we're on first base. Now we've got to figure out, 'Why did we get from homeplate to first base?' *What* immune responses? And then once we learn that, I think we can start to try to push to second base, third base, homeplate.

Our approach has been this. When we get protein, . . . when we are able to use vaccines like the GP160 that we've used, and we give them to individuals that are already infected and we show that the consequence is that they get sick slower and the virus decreases, then we think those vaccines are important candidates to look at in seronegative individuals. And actually we're beginning to do that. But again it's a stepwise fashion.[15]

Unfortunately, the virus has the ability to alter its shape. Once it changes shape, it may be back to the drawing board for a new vaccine. HIV can mutate at a very fast rate, making the genetic diversity of the virus throughout the world more extensive than initially thought. By 1991, more than one hundred HIV-1 isolates had been identified from ten countries on four continents, and in 1989 French researchers discovered what may be a much more virulent form of HIV-1, far more powerful and contagious than either HIV-I or HIV-II. In fact, *all* HIV infected people are apparently infected with several mutant forms of the virus.

HIV can change shape in subtle ways in the same person over the course of a few months, and a person can be infected with several differently shaped viruses at once, possibly with varying abilities to cause disease. Even worse, HIV occasionally changes its shape radically. We are currently seeing new HIV-like viruses emerging every year or two somewhere in the world. There are probably at least four [1988 figure; now some estimate fifteen] HIV-like viruses already. An increasing number of people are infected with more than one type of HIV. Every time someone is infected, there is a minute chance that radical new changes will occur. As the number of infected people worldwide continues to double each year, so does the risk of new strains emerging. Incidentally, most of our tests for infection are for the earliest virus type found. The others can be missed.[16]

Dr. Dixon continues: "The common cold virus is also unstable. That is why we are always getting colds. I probably have antibodies in my blood now to 50 or 100 different shaped cold viruses. By the time one of those viruses has infected people between here, North America, Japan, Korea, India, Greece, and back again, its shape has changed so much that I can catch the same cold all over again. That is why we are light years away from a vaccine against the common cold."[17]

We know today that AIDS is transmitted as a virus particle in blood, semen, pre-seminal fluid, and vaginal fluids, which have been found to contain high concentrations of HIV in infected persons. Whereas it initially enters the helper T-cell, when the cell bursts, large numbers of HIV are released and also become free virus particles traveling throughout the body. But the fact that helper T-cells carry the virus is key. This cell is the immune system's "scavenger" white blood cell and is well suited for carrying the virus to other cells in the body. Unfortunately, "one new study found that macrophages may directly infect rectal cells and cervical cells. Such findings mean the virus can infect partners in anal or vaginal intercourse without any breaks or tears in the skin. Macrophages are present in the blood, the brain, mucous membranes, semen, and cervical fluid."[18]

Further, on March 7, 1988, William Masters and Virginia Johnson held a press conference in New York City to announce the findings in their book *Crisis: Heterosexual Behavior in the Age of AIDS*. Besides documenting rises in heterosexual infection, they alleged that "under rare circumstances the virus could be spread by mosquitoes, . . . dining in restaurants, or using toilet seats."[19] They warn that "deep kissing is another potential means of transmitting the virus and should be avoided."[20]

THE AIDS EPIDEMIC

Without a vaccine or cure, sooner or later AIDS could affect hundreds of millions of people.

- AIDS is now the ninth leading cause of death among children ages one to four and the sixth in ages fifteen to twenty-four. Between 1981 and 1987, AIDS deaths increased a hundredfold. According to Congressional and other studies just released, cases among teenagers are up 77 to 100 percent in the last two years, and AIDS is "spreading unchecked" among young people.[21]

- By 2002 A.D., 60 to 120 million people may be infected with HIV worldwide, 14 million of them in the U.S.[22] That means vastly more Americans will have died from AIDS than from all the wars in our nation's history. The CDC estimates that eight to ten million people are now infected worldwide; however, these figures are probably low because of possible ten-year incubation rates and the "negative window" period of up to fourteen months where a person may have AIDS but cannot yet be diagnosed by testing. The *Los Angeles Times* (February 17, 1991) cited U.S. Census Bureau figures forecasting seventy million cases of AIDS by 2015 in countries south of the Sahara Desert *alone*.[23]

- Several thousand U.S. cases and (apparently) literally millions worldwide have no identifiable risk factor. This means we simply don't know how these people got the disease.[24] In other words, that the virus could be transmitted in ways not yet officially acknowledged cannot be ruled out.

- HIV is a unique and marvelously adaptive/parasitic retrovirus that has an incredible capacity to mutate and prove resistant to medicines. (That is why even AZT is "effective" for an average of only two years.)

- Although now a predominantly homosexual disease in America, it is principally a heterosexual disease in many countries throughout the world, such as Africa and Thailand, where infection rates are much worse than in the U.S. For example, some authorities have recently stated that conditions in Africa are so bad that the battle against AIDS and for Africa has now been lost. Thus, AIDS is not a homosexual disease; it is a viral disease related predominantly to sexual promiscuity—homosexual or heterosexual. The possibility remains that in America the disease could become as widespread among heterosexuals as homosexuals. According to a special program on AIDS on "Dateline NBC" (April 14, 1992) the same tragedy in Africa could happen just as easily in America—and probably will if people do not change their sexual behavior and proper measures are not taken to curtail the spread of AIDS.

- Bisexuals, intravenous drug users, and prostitutes will also increase infection rates among heterosexuals in the U.S. AIDS is rising sharply among women—they now constitute 11 to 15 percent of all U.S. cases—and AIDS is now the fifth leading cause of death among women fifteen to forty-four years old.[25] According to a CNN news report (November 30, 1990) half of all women who die of AIDS didn't even know they were HIV infected.

- AIDS can be spread in at least five different bodily mediums— blood, semen, vaginal secretions, breast milk, and placenta (mother to child). Also, it has been found in saliva, tears, urine, and cerebrospinal fluid, and may possibly exist in several other bodily secretions.[26] Whether it is currently transmitted in these mediums, even rarely, is debated. But even deep kissing, in very rare cases, may have transmitted the virus,[27] and skin is not, apparently, a 100 percent foolproof barrier to transmission.[28]

Another possibility, called the cofactor theory, must be considered. Does HIV by *itself* cause AIDS? There is a small group of scientists who have formed a committee to reassess the role of HIV in the production of AIDS. They maintain that HIV positivity does not necessarily mean that a person will develop the disease. These scientists suggest that a person who gets AIDS after HIV exposure, has probably already been exposed to certain cofactors that will trigger it. These include (1) conditions that compromise the immune system and (2) the presence of certain bacteria and other viruses. Things that compromise the immune system may include a wide variety of sexually transmitted diseases, I.V. drug use, exposure to hepatitis B, pneumonia, tuberculosis, malnutrition, and even having had the stresses involved with multiple blood transfusions through surgery.

In other words, it is individuals who have been in bad shape before exposure to HIV who are most likely to get AIDS as a result of HIV infection. Exposure to any single cofactor, including HIV, will not necessarily kill a person, but the more cofactors a person has, the greater the risk of developing AIDS after HIV exposure.

Because at least 1 percent, and perhaps up to 5 percent, of those diagnosed with AIDS have not yet shown HIV positivity, these scientists argue that one may get AIDS without HIV.

According to this view then, what causes AIDS, at least in America, is *specific* sexual practice or drug use in conjunction with specific *corisk* factors such as immune suppression. Thus, it predominates among the homosexual population because their risk factors are so high (e.g., extensive drug use, anal intercourse, and the presence of widespread STDs). AIDS is common among drug users because drug abuse has also suppressed their immune systems. In similar fashion, it is epidemic in parts of the third world because malnutrition and other factors have suppressed the immune system of additional millions, making them more susceptible to HIV.

Although the cofactor theory is a minority view among scientists, and probably doubtful, it is always possible there may be some truth to it. At the 1992 international AIDS conference it was disclosed that a number of people were diagnosed with AIDS without HIV, indicating either (1) a new virus, which we think is probable, or (2) that we simply don't have all the answers. Further, some studies have apparently indicated that in very rare cases HIV positive people can become HIV/antibody negative and become healthy again. No one knows why. The simple fact is that there are still many things we don't know about the AIDS situation and therefore more discoveries are likely to be made.

The conclusion still holds that HIV and AIDS are sexually transmissible, but it is at least conceivable that there are other factors working besides sexual transmission. If this is so, the non-HIV factors responsible for immunosuppression that might be co-causes of AIDS along with HIV include promiscuous anal intercourse, drug abuse, multiple concurrent infections (hepatitis, STDs, etc.), prolonged high-dose antibiotics, malnutrition due to poverty, alcoholism, and, in theory, anything that would seriously suppress the immune system where HIV is present.

What must be stressed is that this cofactor theory does not lessen the seriousness of the AIDS situation in any respect; it merely addresses the issue of co-causes. AIDS will continue to be a plague in the modern world. If, as some scientists maintain, we have yet to discover the true ramification of how the HIV virus is spread, or that there may be new viruses emerging, the situation could get worse.

In 1981 the reported number of American AIDS cases was less than a few hundred. In February of 1988 the total reported number was 55,167.[29] By November 1989 there were more than 100,000 confirmed cases, with 60,000 dead.[30] By 1993 more than 160,000 had died. Look again at these figures, noting the dates and ratio of infected cases to deaths.

The sad message is that AIDS is an entirely preventable disease. If homosexuals and drug abusers would stop their activities and if heterosexuals would practice celibacy or restrict their sex to an uninfected monogamous relationship, AIDS would stop *dead* in its tracks at current infection rates.

But unfortunately, given current policies things may get worse before they get better. Myron Essex, M.D., Chairman of the Department of Cancer Biology at the Harvard School of Public Health, made the following statement before Congress more than five years ago:

> The Centers for Disease Control have been trying to inform the public without overly alarming them. But we outside the government are freer to speak. The fact is that the dire predictions ever since AIDS appeared haven't been far off the mark. There isn't just one AIDS virus but a score that we know-of—and countless others, because it mutates at a hundred times the rate of other viruses. (*Congressional Record*, March 12, 1986 [S2509 and 2510])

Ward Cates, M.D., of the Centers for Disease Control, stated: "Anyone who has the least ability to look into the future can already see the potential for this disease being much worse than anything mankind has seen before."[31] (See note 31 for more information.)

With the recent Harvard University report estimating that between 30 and 110 million adults and 10 million children worldwide will be HIV infected in the next seven or eight years, who can deny it? Without significant changes in sexual behavior and public policy, before long every one of us will have our own "horror story" to relate concerning AIDS from an acquaintance, friend, or loved one— perhaps even ourselves. Further, the fact that official estimates of future infection rates vary so dramatically indicates that no one really knows what is going on. It is almost as if we are *all* caught up in a gigantic game of Russian roulette. We know the bullet is in the chamber; what we don't know is how long we will decide to play the game.

SUMMARIZING THE PROBLEM

The problem of AIDS is exacerbated by at least five considerations:

1. *No government will risk national panic, widespread vigilantism, and lawlessness if it can avoid these by restricting information.* This has been done in the past and will be done in the future because social order is in the best interests of society. The degree to which information has been restricted in the case of AIDS is anybody's guess, but there is a good possibility that AIDS is of much greater concern to the government than the public suspects. Dr. Dixon discusses eight different areas in which a cover-up of data is being implemented. "A rapidly spreading, silent killer which is difficult to detect, infectious, and lethal causes panic. Radiation disasters are similar: you cannot hear, see, feel or touch the enemy, nor feel the damage it is doing until too late—sometimes not for years."[32]

   Regardless, "cover-up or no cover-up, honesty, secrecy, or confusion, one thing is clear: nothing will ever be quite the same again. AIDS will fundamentally alter fashions, behavior, culture—in fact every fiber of our society."[33] It is no understatement that AIDS will dominate the rest of our adult lives.

2. *Officially, AIDS is believed to be transmitted almost exclusively by contaminated sexual fluids and blood.* The virus resides in these mediums. Hence vaginal or anal intercourse, intravenous drug use, or any activity that transfers contaminated fluids from one body into another, as in unsafe blood transfusions and oral sex, may transmit the disease.

   But various other factors increase susceptibility. For example, a report given at the Fourth International Conference on AIDS in Stockholm (June 12–16, 1988) indicated, "Herpes infection was linked . . . to increased susceptibility to infection by the AIDS virus."[34] As noted earlier, some forty million Americans have herpes. In fact, untreated STDs such as gonorrhea "greatly increase" the chance of contracting AIDS.[35]

   But again, no one is entirely certain that AIDS, in some cases, is not transmitted in other ways. It only appears to be the case today—tomorrow may tell another story. Because the virus is unpredictable and highly mutinagenic no one knows how many new strains will be mutated and whether or not these will be capable of more widespread transmission. According to Dr. Lorraine Day and others, there are rare cases of documented transmission by half a dozen additional methods.[36] The Public Health Service and the former U.S. Surgeon General have gone to great lengths to insist that these are ungrounded fears. But do they really know? Further, are they telling us all they know? And how certain are they about the future?

"Currently, the AIDS pathogen appears to be of low infectivity, but one cannot be sanguine about the trillions of replications of the retrovirus that occur every day in the ever growing host of homosexual carriers. Will one of these replications be a mutation that will 'jump' into the heterosexual community and lay waste immunologically normal bodies? If this disease did not have a vocal constituency is there any doubt that carriers would have been quarantined by now? Dr. John Seale, world known VD expert, has noted, 'If . . . we wait perhaps 20 years before we take drastic preventative action, half the population of the Western World will be wiped out.'"[37]

3. *In deference to the demands of the powerful homosexual lobby (e.g., the National Gay Task Force) no one is keeping accurate records of either partners or infection rates.*[38] Militant homosexual lobbies are doing all in their power to (1) prevent testing, (2) promote their lifestyle as a civil *right*, and (3) disseminate misinformation to the public. What this means is: (1) the official figure of infected is at best an educated guess; the real figures could already be at ten to twenty million; (2) the disease will continue to spread as long as people refuse to change their behavior. Incredibly, the law may even prohibit doctors from informing the partners of an AIDS carrier that he or she has AIDS. If most people with AIDS do not know they have the disease and they continue to spread it, one can only guess at future infection rates. (The best solution to the problem is universal testing. Contrary to stated objections, this would not be inordinately difficult or expensive to achieve—to the contrary, in the long run, it would save a great deal in both money and lives.) In his foreword to the text, *AIDS: The Unnecessary Epidemic*, AIDS authority Stanley Monteith, M.D., warns:

> When historians of the future record the history of this [AIDS] epidemic, they will record a story of malice and mistakes, illusion and delusion, deceit and deception, of dying and death. They will record how the liberal media, highly placed government officials and the U.S. Public Health Service worked in collusion to deceive the American public and convince them that every effort was being made to monitor and control the spread of the disease when, in truth, exactly the opposite was the case.

4. *Most people are not changing their sexual habits:* (1) teenagers are continuing to engage in sex in unprecedented numbers—witness the fact that one-third of all abortions continue to come from teens; (2) many homosexuals may be reducing the number of sexual partners, but not all are. Regardless, the number of sex partners remaining is more than sufficient to continue spread of the disease. So-called "monogamous" relations among homosexuals are rare. Sexual habits in this nation may have already spread the disease among much of the sexually active adult population.

5. *A person is classified as having AIDS only when the "end stage" signs are present* (certain pneumonias, rare tumors, and so on). Unfortunately, this is rather like diagnosing someone with cancer only after years of chemotherapy and when they have only three months to live. The truth almost exclusively is that from the point of infection a person has the death sentence of AIDS. Current classification methods may keep the number of infected low, but they are also misleading.

ADDENDUM:
ADDITIONAL DATA ABOUT AIDS

- In Buddhist Thailand 90 percent of the men have had sex with a prostitute by the age of nineteen; that means there will be up to four million dead in Thailand alone in the next eight years. The nation's gigantic tourist sex market has also helped spread AIDS throughout the world. AIDS is so bad in Thailand that a leader in the fight against it told American men on television, "Why do you come over here and have sex with the prostitutes? Why don't you just stay there and eat rat poison—it's cheaper."[39]

- In America and France one half or more of all hemophiliacs are now innocent victims of AIDS.

- In Africa, some estimate 50 to 70 percent of the population over fifteen years of age may be infected with HIV—up to 150 million people. In the end, AIDS may have destroyed an entire continent. Who can possibly calculate such a cost?

- The AIDS virus seems to be more resilient than first thought; it is not killed by alcohol after twenty minutes of immersion and can survive outside the body for more than a week.[40] In some cases, the AIDS virus stays alive and infective on a dry surface at room temperature for seven days.[41]

- Condoms are less safe than originally thought. Condoms fail 14.2 percent of the time when used to prevent pregnancy. "So the 14.2 percent figure for pregnancy could theoretically be doubled, tripled or quadrupled for transmission of HIV even with the use of condoms"—because while women can become pregnant only three to four days per month, AIDS can be transmitted every day of the month.[42]

- Surgical gloves are less safe than originally thought.[43]

- A single needle prick can transmit the AIDS virus.[44]

- The experts are constantly revising their opinions on AIDS because of constantly emerging new information.[45] "The need to make such revisions has eroded health care authorities' status as experts. The appearance of having 'changed their minds' again and again has crippled their credibility and undermined efforts at reassurance."[46]

- One target cell for the AIDS virus may be in the intact skin: "The assumption that HIV infection occurs exclusively by the entry of virus through wounds in skin and mucous membranes into the blood can no longer be considered valid. Our results suggest that the Langerhans cells in the skin and mucous membranes are the primary target cells for sexually transmitted HIV infection." [47]

- Only a single HIV particle can be infective.[48]

- Sexual partners cannot be trusted for AIDS protection. For instance, "Of 90 men and women known to be infected with HIV, 45 continue to have sex. All of the women who continue to have sex inform their partners of their HIV status. Seventeen men continue to have sex without informing their partners."[49]

- AIDS may be transmitted in certain cases by saliva.[50] Further, "forty-five couples were tested showing that 91 percent had blood in their saliva after deep kissing."[51]

- AIDS patients are increasingly contracting resilient forms of tuberculosis, greatly raising the risk of contamination of hospital workers and also the general public.[52]
- HIV infection can be produced in aerosols generated by power instruments in the operating room: "Surgeons are not being tested routinely for HIV, so no one knows how many are positive, and it will take four to seven years for surgeons to develop full-blown AIDS and become sick."[53] Dr. Day reveals, "I personally know of 17 surgeons who are infected with the AIDS virus from occupational exposure, eight of whom are orthopedic surgeons. I know of five non-surgeon doctors who are positive from needlesticks. . . . They haven't told their superiors."[54]

The following are excerpted from Patrick Dixon's *The Whole Truth About AIDS*. Dixon (M.A., Cambridge University; M.D., London University) is director of AIDS Care Education and Training, specializing in volunteer help for people with AIDS. He has lived in Africa and the U.S. and recently visited San Francisco and Central Africa to see firsthand the AIDS disasters there.

- "In Edinburgh, Scotland, the virus has spread from one addict to infect between one thousand and two thousand other people in 18 months" (p. 63).[55]
- "Half of the people with AIDS will develop signs of brain impairment or nerve damage during their illness" (p. 57). Apparently, many AIDS patients are dying of unknown causes suspected of being related to AIDS but never diagnosed as such.[56]
- In New York, AIDS is now the most common cause of death in women aged twenty-five to thirty-four; further, one in every sixty-one babies carries the virus (p. 18).
- Thousands of people have been dying of AIDS for years, but their deaths were blamed on other diseases (p. 18).
- In some parts of Central Africa up to 20 percent of all young women and their babies are believed to be infected; entire villages are being wiped out; in some hospitals, between 8 and 23 percent of the blood supply is infected (p. 18).

- "Right now HIV is spreading like wildfire through communities of drug addicts in the United States, to their husbands, wives, lovers, children, and out into the wider community" (p. 19).
- An American study indicated that 70 percent of gay men reported having sex with a woman in the previous three to four years (p. 19).
- Children can become infected from being molested by infected fathers; organ transplants have also infected people (p. 22).
- Incredibly, some have claimed that up to one-third of all fifty-seven thousand Roman Catholic priests could be infected with AIDS (p. 22).
- One or 2 percent of HIV carriers *never* produce a positive test. In other words, of every 10 million infected individuals, 100,000 to 200,000 are permanent silent spreaders (p. 27). Of course, the millions who refuse to be tested are also silent spreaders.[59]
- In September 1988 the Red Cross admitted that it released more than 2,400 suspect blood products. In addition, "the security of the system is jeopardized by technicians who borrow secret pass codes to erase or alter records. In one region, a computer automatically labeled blood as safe even though hepatitis tests were never performed. In another, records of more than 24,000 collections [of blood] were lost (p. 37).

But, there are even more serious things to consider.

1. *Cases of deliberate infection or apparent "revenge" sex are increasing.* In Michigan, an infected homosexual knowingly had sex with hundreds of teenage boys.[60]

An AIDS patient received ten years in prison and was found guilty of attempted murder for biting a policeman.[61]

A boy prostitute in London was taken into custody because of his deliberate attempts to infect others with AIDS.[62]

A drug addict in Norway "infected fifty people after he discovered he had the disease [AIDS]."[63]

A drug addict was jailed for three years for spitting in a policeman's eyes "to give him AIDS."[64]

2. *Thousands of physicians and health care workers may die in the near future:* "Just how many people will need medical care for AIDS over the next 20 years? Millions. Maybe 75 million in Africa alone.

Even if the risk [to health care workers] from an individual patient is small, the risk can be multiplied millions of times. The fact is that a large number of doctors and nurses worldwide are going to die of AIDS over the next decade or two unless there is a cure or a vaccine."[65]

3. *AIDS may have already spread rapidly throughout the heterosexual population.* It requires little calculation to realize that hundreds of thousands of silent carriers can easily infect millions of others. Women become infected from men both with and without using condoms. Most homosexuals are bisexual, further complicating the spread into the heterosexual population. For example, many homosexuals are also married. "To be precise and accurate, most people who call themselves homosexual should more correctly be self identified as bisexual."[66]

Unfortunately, the spread of AIDS by prostitutes and drug abusers into the general population is at least, if not more, serious than from bisexuals.[67]

The foregoing is only a small indication of the AIDS story. What no one can deny is that we are faced with a nightmare.

The Myth of "Consenting Adults"

The Social Cost of Current
Sexual Attitudes

The mounting evidence indicting the leaders of the sexual revolution is impressive. They promised joy, liberation, and good health. They've delivered misery, disease and even death.

Vernon Mark, M.D.

One of the prevailing myths of our time is the idea that sex between consenting adults (or teens) is no one else's business. Despite the fact that all civilized societies have done so for millennia, we are told that it is "wrong," "bigoted," and "intolerant" to assume the right to tell anyone else how he or she should live. Planned Parenthood, leading talk show hosts/news commentators, politicians, and others tell us that not only is it none of our business, it is also none of the government's business what an individual does with his private sex life. Further, it is not the school's business, parents' business, or the church's business. To teach others to restrict their sexual behavior is supposedly "puritanical," "harmful," and "repressive."

But more and more people are beginning to realize that they do suffer personally from the sexual actions of others. The economic cost of AIDS and other sexually transmitted diseases alone will be in the hundreds of *billions* of dollars—and all of us will pay for it—including our children and their children.

Some people don't yet realize that their diminishing health coverage (at significantly higher rates) is increasingly due to the nation's continued acceptance of homosexuality and its cost in AIDS—as well as other massive financial costs of the sexual revolution. This does not even consider the emotional and social costs.

McDowell is absolutely correct when he warns,

> A "private act" of illicit sex can have widespread and horrendous physical, social, political, economical, emotional and moral implications for the society which condones it. Historically, those groups which originated legislation to regulate the sexual activities of a given culture were not primarily religious, such as the Puritans. It was often secular governments who had the common sense to realize that sex is not only a private act, but also one with potentially appalling public consequences and costs. Someone always pays for promiscuity—and it is not always the primary participants who pay the most.[1]

Some of the most horrible tragedies are those forced upon the innocent:

- infants and children
- hemophiliacs
- a faithful spouse
- teenagers who will die young

McDowell proceeds to point out that it costs federal and state governments an average of $100,000 in medical and welfare costs for every teen who has a child—and each year 1.2 million teenagers get pregnant. In just the year of 1985, teenage childbearing cost the nation more than $16 billion.[2]

It is estimated that in the next twenty years American taxpayers will pay well in excess of $100 *billion* for the net results of teenage pregnancies alone.[3] As McDowell points out, that is an exceptionally large sum for the public to have to pay for so-called private acts.

It is anyone's guess how much AIDS will cost the American public in the next twenty years. The estimated cost of AIDS in New York alone from 1989 to 1994 is 7 or 8 billion.[4] For the rest of the country, estimates vary between $5 and $15 billion per year. The amount spent on other sexually transmitted diseases is equally staggering—in the multiple billions[5]—not to mention all the parallel consequences and ramifications of these diseases.

By the year 2010 the total cost could be $1,000 to $5,000 *billion* —and probably more—for the consequences of promiscuous sex, including abortion, AIDS and other STDs, welfare, medical costs, psychological counseling, lost productivity, increased health insurance premiums, prison terms, court fees, legal defense, rape and child abuse, and so on. (Some have even spoken in terms of a quadrillion dollars—a thousand trillion dollars—before this is all over.) A recent study by the Society of Actuaries estimated that AIDS itself would cost national insurance companies more than $100 billion in life, health, and disability claims merely by the year 2000.[6] In light of such figures, let us ask some questions.[7]

If it is none of our business what anyone else does with his or her sex life, why do we have to pay for it? If private acts of sex are no one else's concern, why do we all pay billions for AIDS research, "family planning," abortion, pregnancy counseling, and all the rest?

If American citizens will pay billions or trillions of dollars for the "private acts" of consenting adults and teenagers, why don't the promiscuous even want us to find out whether or not they have the AIDS virus and are freely spreading it to others? How can they logically demand the collective right to continue to practice sexual activity that is destroying millions of lives and then turn around and demand that society care and pay for the victims of their own behavior?

Why are homosexual groups everywhere, Planned Parenthood, and other sexually active pressure groups asking for millions of dollars for public school sex education beginning in the first grade?

Why should the public fund abortions when it is the sexual irresponsibility of the partners that produced the pregnancy? When the money is not available, why should the public care for victims of AIDS and other STDs when they had nothing to do with it?

When a husband commits adultery against his wife, and then gives her AIDS, do her husband's private acts have no consequences on her personal life? If it is possible for a person to be a carrier of HIV and other STDs for several years without knowing it, and if sex with any given person is now sex with every person that person had sex with—how is this no one else's business?

Consider how gonorrhea and syphilis typically spread. This happens to be a true story: A girl had sex with sixteen different men. The men then had sex with other women who had sex with other men who had sex with other women, and so on. The number of traced contacts finally added up to 1,660![8] Unfortunately, the same thing is happening worldwide with the AIDS virus—and again, most of those who are being infected don't even *know* it.

All this means that sex is no longer a private act when the sexually promiscuous demand that the American public spend billions of dollars to care for and attempt to cure their own willfully chosen diseases.

But pay we will! For some sixty sexually transmitted diseases, single parents' welfare costs, AIDS, and perhaps millions of babies born with the diseases inherited from the sexual activity of their parents. In 1991 PID alone was costing $4 billion a year to treat.[9]

Unfortunately, the emotional toll is often worse than the physical or financial toll. Consider the more than, 160,000 Americans who have already died of AIDS and the emotional wreckage it has left in the lives of their families and friends.

After one of his speaking engagements, Josh McDowell was approached by a woman who was nearly hysterical. She explained to McDowell that she had been married for four years to a man who had been in excellent health. One day he was informed he had AIDS—twelve days later he was dead. The disease was traced back to an affair he had six years earlier.[10] What's worse, the physicians told this woman that she had to be tested every three months for the next several years. Place yourself in this woman's shoes. How would you feel? She can't sleep nights. She finds it difficult to concentrate at work. All the while, she is tormented with the idea that she will one day test positive and, like her husband, die. Then what will happen? Who will care for her children? Who will care for her aging parents?

This woman has paid a high price for one "private act" of her husband's. Now multiply this situation by the millions and you may begin to see the social magnitude of the problem.

How do you build trust in a marriage or other relationship when one partner infects another with AIDS, gonorrhea, PID, herpes, chlamydia, or syphilis? Do we have any idea how many men visit prostitutes every year in this country? It numbers in the millions. Incredibly, many of them are married. "The average prostitute in the United States has had sex with 2,000 men. That man just didn't have a private act of sex with a prostitute. He had sex with the prostitute, plus her 2,000 partners, plus all of their partners for the past ten years—up to 12,000 people. Then, that man has the audacity to go home and have sex with his wife! His wife didn't have a private act in bed with her husband. She had sex with her husband, plus the prostitute, plus her 2,000 partners, plus all their partners for the last ten years. That's a lot to handle as a wife."[11]

But there are also costs for young people to pay for the "private acts" of others. Parents must now explain to their children something that parents of any other generation have never had to do—nor could they have ever imagined such a thing. Parents today must soberly tell their own children that they cannot have peace of mind on their wedding night or at any point afterward unless they know certain information. They must know the detailed sexual history of their mate and all their mate's partners for the past ten years. They must know this information with absolute accuracy—or risk death.

Even young children pay by becoming infected with HIV and other STDs. There are already millions of such children, and in the future there could be more. Many of these children will suffer with moderate to serious physical diseases from nonfatal STDs and a good percentage of them will pay with their own lives when they contract a fatal STD like AIDS. One hospital reports that the lifetime care cost for children with AIDS averages more than $90,000 per child.[12] Various researchers in Europe and America have revealed that up to 25 to 40 percent of newborns to mothers infected with AIDS are themselves infected with the virus.[13]

Then consider all the children who have one or more parents dying from AIDS. They too pay a terrible price. We earlier cited World Health Organization estimates that by 2002 almost thirty *million* children will be orphaned by AIDS.

According to several sources, more than thirty thousand single mothers with AIDS in New York, having an average of two children, will die by 1995, leaving the city to attempt to provide for sixty thousand foster children.[14] That's sixty thousand children whose mothers have died of AIDS, many of whom themselves are at risk. The human cost, physically and emotionally, is unimaginable.

Then, of course, we haven't even considered the other innocent victims of AIDS, such as hemophiliacs—tens of thousands more who are cruelly given a death sentence because of the "private acts" of others.

Now consider a final illustration of such "private acts"—abortion. Some thirty million unborn children in America alone have already paid the ultimate price for their parents' sexual irresponsibility—being killed while yet in a mother's womb. Worldwide, the figure is around one-half *billion.*

How long God might put up with all this, no one knows, but anyone who claims that the private sexual life of another person is none of your business is either uninformed or lying. Yet the myth of "private consent" persists.

In *What's Wrong with Sex Education?* Melvin Anchell warns, "To stop the destruction of our civilization, America must re-establish its social conscience."[15] To illustrate, on "The Geraldo Show" of October 19, 1991, a panel of women were presented who had been engaging in sexual acts with family members. Even when a sister was having sex with her own brother, several people in the audience began their statement with "I have no right to tell you you are wrong but . . ." When many Americans don't even have the conviction to say *incest* is wrong, how will the nation ever say infidelity and the more common forms of sexual promiscuity are wrong?

Think about the following list of sexually related issues—from pornography and child molestation to infertility and prostitution (with its "acceptable" level of crime and drugs)—what do you think is the final physical, emotional, fiancial and spiritual cost represented in all these activities?

- Sexual dysfunction and the counseling it requires
- Teenage pregnancy
- Incest
- Sexual child abuse by parents, siblings, neighbors, and strangers
- Adultery and divorce
- Surrogate sex therapy (e.g., therapists who have sex with clients, both married and single, to help them perform better or eradicate their sexual problems)
- Abortion
- Psychological problems: personal guilt, depression, low self-esteem, even suicide induced by illicit sexual activity, abortion, divorce, and so on.
- Sadomasochistic sex
- Homosexuality and lesbianism
- Sixty sexually transmitted diseases
- Prostitution—male, female, child
- AIDS
- Single parenthood
- Rape
- Pornography
- Snuff films/bestiality

Consider the following additional data:

1. Thanks largely to AIDS, cases of tuberculosis are exploding around the country. *Newsweek* warned, "Without prompt action, TB could decimate some segments of society."[16]
2. Ten to 30 percent of children born to AIDS-infected parents are infected and will die by age four without treatment, but treatment is so costly society cannot afford it. Hospital costs aside, even AIDS home health care can require up to $25,000 per month.
3. In the U.S. alone $10 to $12 billion per year will be spent on AIDS from 1993 to 1995. Then costs will escalate. In just the next five years, costs may increase tenfold. This means a community now paying $10 million a year for AIDS treatment will be paying $100 million a year.
4. Unfortunately, these expenses seem to have occurred at the point where researchers were close to perhaps dramatic breakthroughs in several serious illnesses, including heart disease and cancer. Because of the vast sums of money spent on sexually related illness, these breakthroughs will either be delayed for decades or never realized simply because the money that would have been available was not. Because HIV is the first virus in history having powerful civil protections, the money spent on curing it is disproportional. For example, the *Journal of the American Family Association* reported that heart disease now claims twenty times more lives than AIDS, yet receives only one-third of its funding. Cancer claims thirteen times more lives and receives only 90 percent of AIDS funding. Diabetes and Alzheimers together claim three times the deaths of AIDS yet receive only about 13 percent of its budget. The injustice is not that so much is spent on AIDS, for it is a potentially more serious disease. The problem is that society encouraged the very conditions that gave rise to a disease that otherwise might never have existed—and at the expense of other medical research.[17]
5. By the turn of the century, we will have spent scores or hundreds of dollars on sexually related diseases, illnesses, and their consequences—money that could have been far more profitably spent elsewhere.

Is an individual's sexual behavior really nobody else's business?

8

The Media's Prejudicial Ethics

Is There an Entrenched Bias Against the Moral Absolutes That Would Stop Sexual Plagues?

John Weldon remembers several discussions he had with certain professors while an undergraduate in the turbulent 1960s. What characterized those academics was their promotion of liberal sexual attitudes and their corresponding dislike for Christian values. Some of the comments, in and out of the classroom, included: "Christianity is a myth for insecure people"; "Jesus Christ is the figment of a psychotic imagination"; "Only a fool would be a Christian"; "What the world needs is a humanistic approach to life that rejects Christian standards"; and "Christians who promote absolutist values upon society are suffering from an unhealthy fear of sexuality instituted by an archaic biblical standard."

These comments were made more than twenty years ago. Today, the dividing line between those few who accept moral absolutes and the majority who reject them is stronger than ever. It illustrates the major cause of the current sexual tragedy stalking our nation.

Masters and Johnson emphasize, "There is no sexual value system that is right for everyone and no single moral code that is indisputably correct and universally applicable."[1] Such a statement reflects the current bias in American culture against Christian values, in particular, absolute moral values. Consider the recent history of such organizations as Planned Parenthood, People for the American Way, the ACLU, and even the national Democratic Party. Such organizations are largely secularist institutions that oppose Christian values and that, because of their opposition, can harm the general health of the public.

These organizations are frequently prohomosexual and pro-abortion; they use their political platform or other power in support of sexual perversion and the murder of the unborn. They characteristically reject moral absolutes and encourage, directly or indirectly, the very kinds of thinking and behavior that will result in millions of deaths from sexually transmitted diseases.

Indeed, on the eve of President Bush's August 1992 acceptance speech, NBC nightly news commentator John Chancellor emphasized the he did not want moral leadership coming from the president of the United States. One can only wonder when respected social commentators say such things. Perhaps appropriately, during the same convention, "Queer Nation," a militant homosexual group, vandalized Republican party headquarters, protesting its affirmation of family values as "discriminatory."

In addition, there are the liberal college professors, psychologists, educators, humanists, teachers' unions, pornographers, homosexuals, and militant feminists who are working hard to push their own agenda.[2] Several studies have documented the liberal, humanistic, and anti-Christian bias of those who control the American electronic media (for example, television and movie producers). It is as if the entertainment media has deliberately attempted to sell Americans its own distorted set of values concerning sexuality and other matters. In fact, quite appropriately "Entertainment Tonight" (May 28, 1986) stated in a special segment on the billion dollar pornography industry that some of the industry's financial backers refused to be interviewed because of their prominent positions in the entertainment business.

THE IMPACT OF THE MEDIA

In a special report on television violence, *TV Guide* (August 22, 1992) noted that more than sufficient studies had been done to conclude that violence on television can produce violence in children: "The NIMH [National Institute of Mental Health] states the consensus [of all these studies]: 'Violence on television does lead to aggressive behavior by children and teenagers who watch the programs.'"

Further, it cited Leonard D. Eron and others in "one of the most ambitious and conclusive studies" yet published: "There can no longer be any doubt that heavy exposure to televised violence is one of the causes of aggressive behavior, crime, and violence in society. The evidence comes from both the laboratory and real-life studies. Television violence affects youngsters of all ages, of both genders, at all socio-economic levels, and all levels of intelligence." If movie and television violence causes violent behavior among viewers, on what logical basis can we assume that sexual immorality in movies and television is entirely without impact?

No less an authority than Brandon Tartikoff, former head of Paramount Studios and NBC, observed on "Larry King Live" (October 16, 1992) that "television is a medium that is going to encourage imitation." He warned that networks should be careful to instill some kind of moral values because people's actions *are* influenced by television. (If this is true even for something as terrible as news stories about suicide, it may certainly also be true for television sex. An article in the *New England Journal of Medicine*, 315, no. 11, p. 685, concluded that "television stories about suicide trigger additional suicides, perhaps because of imitation.")

For the most part, sex as portrayed on TV and the movies is not true to life. For example, according to one study, 94 percent of sexual encounters on soap operas were between people not married to one another.[3] In other words, television is telling viewers, including children and teens, that most sex occurs outside of marriage, even though that is not true. The "soaps" constantly tell us that sex is just another casual, fun activity without consequence. "Unfortunately, our society is filled with messages from the media, music and even certain laws (e.g., abortion on demand) that encourage teens to engage in sex in a hedonistic way without acknowledging consequences."[4] A study by Lou Harris and Associates revealed "that 41 percent of teenagers think that television gives a realistic picture of the consequences of sex. What may be even more sobering is that 24 percent of adults believe what they see about sex on TV—one out of four!"[5]

Many people think that children aren't behaviorally influenced by movies, music videos, and television. But that is false. The fact that TV advertisers spend billions of dollars each year on advertising during prime time television reveals the power of the media.

How could it be otherwise, given the time we spend with it? The amount of time the average teenager spends watching TV and listening to music videos is equivalent to the amount of time he spends in school from grade one through four years of college. From grade seven to twelve alone, kids listen to an average total of 10,500 hours of rock music—not even considering the amount of time they spend watching TV.[6] What kinds of messages are portrayed in rock music videos and most TV programs concerning sexual behavior? There are basically three messages: (1) doing what "feels good" or what's "right for you"—which usually translates into sexual permissiveness; (2) the idea that sex is a private act and no one else's business—which leads to sexual irresponsibility; and (3) the belief that sexual behavior is largely without personal consequence —which usually brings personal acts of considerable consequence.

Some research studies have estimated that the average person views more than ninety thousand scenes of sex or suggested sexual intercourse between the ages of eight and eighteen—more than seventy thousand of them involving pre- or extramarital intercourse.[7] Can anyone really believe that ninety thousand scenes of sex or suggested sex has no influence whatever? As one girl who had just lost her virginity wrote us, "I just couldn't compete with what I saw on television; the bombardment never stopped, and so I said, ['What's the difference?']"

The fact that children are being innocently indoctrinated with a liberal view of sex, not to mention the other distortions, has hardly even been protested by parents:

> Many of us share in the blame because of our permissiveness. How much guidance have we given our children about the kinds of television programs and movies to watch? Have we written to our local television stations when they broadcast something we did not approve of? In most cases, I think we have lost the battle without putting up a fight. For years too many of us have been silent about the dangerous effects of media on our kids.[8]

McDowell is convinced that, " 'TV'—the electronic babysitter—has probably done more to shape attitudes of teens than any other single factor of American life, especially with the advent of cable television."[9] A study he cites, "The Impact of Media on the Sexual Attitudes of Adolescents," given to the National Council on Family Relations Annual Conference, revealed that there appeared to be "a correlation between the total media time of the students and their premarital sexual attitudes."[10]

Most studies show that, in order of influence, the three factors molding teenagers' values and behavior are (1) parents, (2) peers, (3) the media (TV, radio, movies).[11] A few studies show the order as (1) peers, (2) media, and (3) parents.[12] The study just cited revealed a strong correlation between the favorite movies of adolescents and their premarital sexual attitudes. According to McDowell, "When youth selected R or X rated movies as their most preferred, the probability that they would have a permissive sexual attitude was extremely high. On the other hand, those who chose PG as most preferred were traditional in their premarital sexual attitudes."[13]

A girl from West Virginia wrote: "I accepted Jesus as my savior when I was nine. I have been going to church all my life and still do. At age seventeen I began dating a boy who had graduated and gotten work with a factory in town. I thought he was cool. Well, one night we went to see the movie *10*. On the way home, we took a detour and had intercourse in the back seat of his mother's car. After five months of dating, he broke up with me. I was crushed."[14]

Considering television and movies as a whole, the number of illicit sexual episodes shown is beyond counting. And networks have either done away with their departments for program standards or reduced their staff.[15] This may be because of the pressure exerted by the success of cable stations—which are increasingly permissive and garnering a larger and larger share of the viewing audience.

What the modern American media tells our children about sex is that everyone is doing it. Today we also have dozens of powerful media personalities—rock stars, TV stars, and movie stars—openly proclaiming their liberal sexual attitudes. If such personalities are our national heroes, why should we think our kids don't listen to them?

THE IRRESPONSIBILITY OF THE MEDIA

"Adult" magazines such as *Cosmopolitan, Mademoiselle,* and *Elle* now carry explicit sexual articles that were once reserved for *Playboy*— and yet many of these magazines are marketed to and read by teenagers and even preteens. A college co-ed wrote to us:

> Reading all these magazines with their detailed articles on the techniques and joys of petting, oral sex, sexual intercourse, etc., made it impossible for me to resist getting involved sexually with my boyfriend. But my getting a sexually transmitted disease and breaking up with Jimmy wasn't the real problem.

I became more and more fascinated with the articles on extramarital affairs. I began having fantasies about what it would be like to have a relationship with a married man. Soon, I had one.

More than anything else in life—major surgery, a broken family, job rejections, worry of AIDS, more than anything else—I will never get over this and what it did. We were caught together in bed at his beach house. His wife didn't just divorce him; she shot him dead. I feel responsible. How am I supposed to live with this?

Further, how many movies, music videos, and magazines actively portray positive moral values? Most of the media continue to glamorize the very activity that will result in the deaths of millions of people.

Why is so much tragedy in real life associated with what is potentially such a wonderful physical act? Perhaps one reason is because sex is far more than merely a physical act; it is always an emotional and spiritual act as well. Second, the most important sex organ is the mind, and when the mind is corrupted, everything else suffers. Third, God never created us with the internal ability to discard His moral law with impunity. But none of this is shown on TV.

Are teenagers or adults ever shown a baby born with birth defects from an STD? Are they shown pictures of people dying with AIDS? Are they ever shown the emotional turmoil in people's lives as a result of casual sex? Are they ever shown the results of an abortion? Despite his endless affairs, did J. R. Ewing on "Dallas" ever get a venereal disease? On other shows, have any of the sexually active movie stars ever done so?

In preparation for this book, we examined several months of programs from popular talk shows, including Oprah, Geraldo, Donahue, Sonya Live, Jenny Jones, Sally Raphael. Consider some of the topics: sexual addictions, adultery, incest, rape, sexual swingers, siblings having sex with their sibling's boyfriends/girlfriends, mothers giving their teenage daughters birth control pills and encouraging them to have sex with boyfriends, phone sex, child prostitutes, parents counseling their pregnant daughters to have abortions, mothers sleeping with their daughters' boyfriends, fathers sleeping with their sons' girlfriends, mothers and daughters sleeping with the same man, lesbianism and lesbian nude bars, homosexuality and various other (even more) perverted forms of sex, pornography, sexual abuse of children, and worse.

Tens of millions of people watch these shows. Should we assume that they are without influence on either adult or teenage behavior? Audience reaction frequently indicates heartfelt support for sexual behavior that is clearly sinful from a Christian perspective. Do these shows do no more than titillate viewers—or are they increasingly a reflection of actual American values?

For two decades, we have permitted the media to distort the consequences of sexual activity. Our children have been shown that casual sex is either a cure for their personal problems of loneliness and low self-esteem or a means to their being successful and making money.

Thus, not only does the secular media not reinforce moral values or demonstrate the consequences of illicit sex, it often actively promotes the opposite. It continues to cultivate feelings of inadequacy among young people. So much emphasis is placed on sex or beauty that children grow up thinking these are the most important aspects of their being. If a woman is not beautiful, she is unimportant. If she doesn't have the right figure, she won't get a man to look at her. How can any child develop a healthy sense of self-worth when the emphasis is on physical standards of perfection, which 90 percent of them will never attain? The same is true for men. Men are supposed to be good looking "studs" who can satisfy all the women they want. Does such an attitude help men become loving husbands and fathers?

And what have our political representatives done in light of the vast consequences of the sexual revolution? Have they supported it or opposed it? Rather than stand for morality, Congress has wasted billions of dollars on special interest groups or its own agenda, helping to force the nation deeper and deeper into the most severe debt of its history. Unfortunately, for the first time in American history a U.S. President now supports both abortion and homosexual rights.

Perhaps an argument can be made that our national attitudes won't change unless the attitudes of those in the media and those who run the country also begin to change.

The Biases of Modern Value-Free Sex Education

What Are They Doing to Our Children?

Jerry, an eighteen year old from a small West Coast town, wrote us the following letter:

> Sex education is great. By the time I was seventeen, I had learned different ways to have sex without engaging in intercourse, several ways to have intercourse but prevent pregnancy, all the positions—and how to avoid all the sexually transmitted diseases. The books told me about how great orgasms are and, in an age of AIDS, how important petting and oral sex are. They were right; they are great. . . .
>
> The school nurse who taught us did her best. She admitted that the only foolproof method for avoiding pregnancy was abstinence, but agreed this method wasn't very practical.
>
> You might be interested in knowing the results. Perhaps we learned that sex ed might not be so great. Five years later, seven of the 18 girls in the class had become pregnant (one married, three are single moms, and three had abortions), eight of us have contracted an STD of one kind or another and one has AIDS. The school nurse was murdered under mysterious circumstances, and the local gay group has pressured the school board to allow their president to teach the class for at least two years. I still think sex ed is necessary, but I don't know if the right message is getting through.

Based on local standards, sex education materials vary across the nation. Some are influenced by homosexual propaganda, some are not. Some actively teach a liberal view of sex, others do not. Concerned individuals need to examine their own children's sex education to determine its approach to human sexuality and the specific content of the courses. Programs that include the following descriptive titles are usually the most suspect: *Value Free, Morally Neutral, Values Clarification, Nondirective Education, Decision-Making Education, Process Education, Affective or Experiential Education,* and even *Self-Esteem Building.* Where the information in such programs is false, biased, scientifically suspect, or physically or emotionally harmful, it should be actively protested by those who are concerned about their children's welfare.

THE FAILURE OF SEX EDUCATION

A number of studies have shown that comprehensive sex education programs do not work and can actually be destructive to the lives of teens and preteens.

Brad Hayton summarizes the results of his own research: "In sum, sex education programs that promote the use of condoms increase teenage pregnancy rates, abortion rates, rates of premarital sex, sexually transmitted diseases, and lower grades and academic aspirations."[1]

Dinah Richard concludes, "Comprehensive sex education, particularly in the form of 'values-neutral' decision making, has been adopted into the classroom. Not only has this not reduced the problem of teenage pregnancy, it has been positively correlated to an increase in adolescent sexual activity, abortion, sexually transmitted diseases, and accompanying psychological problems."[2]

Researchers Joseph Olsen and Stan Weed also documented that greater adolescent involvement in federal family planning programs is associated with significantly higher teenage pregnancy and abortion rates.[3]

> The correlation between funding for family planning and high levels of teen pregnancies and abortions applies not only to federal programs, but to small state programs as well. As revealed in testimony before the U.S. Senate Committee on Labor and Human Resources, those states with the highest expenditures on family planning and with similar socio-demographic characteristics showed the largest increases in abortion and illegitimate births. When comparing selected states to the national average, it becomes glaringly apparent that the rate of teenage pregnancy and abortion closely parallels funding for family planning.[4]

Reviewing studies by family planning groups reveals that despite widespread use of contraceptives, not only are abortions increasing, so are repeat abortions.

> These studies show that even when teens regularly use contraceptives, they can still become pregnant, and that the pregnancies often end in abortion. Rather than curtailing sexual activity, many of the same teens re-enter the cycle, resulting in repeated pregnancies and repeated abortions. Notwith-

standing, advocates of family planning do not see (or acknowledge) that their programs are failures. In fact, some advocates justify abortion as a necessary means of fertility control when contraceptives fail. As the Guttmacher Institute stated in its 1981 report . . . the decline in births is largely contingent on continued access to legal abortions.[5]

In *Sex and Pregnancy in Adolescence* researchers Zelnik and Kantner confess that there was an "almost total absence of evidence" for any benefits of comprehensive sex education.[6] Further, "a review of thirty-three studies of sex education showed that there were gains in sexual knowledge, but shifts toward more liberal sexual attitudes, which led to promiscuity."[7]

In the March 1989 issue of *Pediatrics*, Dr. James W. Stout reviewed five studies on the effects of sex education and concluded that sex education has had little impact on altering sexual activity, promoting the use of birth control, or lowering teenage pregnancy. . . . A study of sex education by Johns Hopkins University [concluded] . . . 'The final result to emerge from the analysis is that neither pregnancy education nor contraceptive education exerts any significant effect on the risk of premarital pregnancy among sexually active teenagers—finding that calls into question the argument that formal sex education is an effective tool for reducing adolescent pregnancy.' . . . What contemporary educators fail to realize is that the boldness of their approach seems to desensitize young people and inclines them to become more permissive. That finding goes all the way back to the very first sex education program in the Western world—the Swedish approach. In 1956, when Sweden mandated sex education, the illegitimacy rate, which had been declining, rose for every school age group, except the older ones, who did not receive the special education. The same can be said about sex education in American schools."[8]

Not surprisingly, the majority of four hundred randomly selected family physicians and psychiatrists also agreed that the availability of teenage contraceptives had led to an increase in promiscuity.[9]

All this is why proponents of sex education who cite studies "proving" its alleged benefits in reducing teenage pregnancy should be viewed with caution. For example, "Planned Parenthood printed a review of studies claiming that sex education was beneficial, but the same studies showed that the teenage promiscuity and pregnancy rates had increased, not decreased, during the time span in question."[10]

THE PROBLEMS OF SEX EDUCATION

But there are other problems associated with modern sex education. For example, it "has also been correlated with an increase in emotional problems for adolescents. Dr. Myre Sim, Professor of Psychiatry at the University of Ottawa, has described the approach used by contemporary sex educators as 'bad education.'"[11]

Psychoanalyst Melvin Anchell warns that "typical sex education courses are almost perfect recipes for producing personality problems and even perversions later in life. . . . Sex education programs from kindergarten through high school continually downgrade the affectionate, monogamous nature of human sexuality."[12]

Young children can easily be harmed by receiving explicit instruction on human sexuality at an age when they are not yet ready for it. Although the nation's sex education curricula are increasingly encouraging sex education to begin with kindergarten, most experts seem to agree that this is not a good idea. Interest in sex is something that usually coincides with puberty, and it is at this point that proper sex education should begin. Before this stage, it may only arouse dormant feelings and actually lead to sexual activity. "The testimonies of experts in child development confirm the dangers of sex education during the latency period [age six through puberty]. Dr. John Meek, Director of Child and Adolescent Services at the Psychiatric Institute of Washington, says, 'It is clear that sexual instruction in the lower elementary grades is unwarranted and potentially destructive to a large percentage of our children.'"[13]

Sean O'Reilly, professor at the School of Medicine and Health Services at George Washington University, claims that detailed sex instruction, whether in a coeducational classroom or in private to prepubertal children is "ill-advised and potentially harmful."[14] Psychoanalyst Rhoda L. Lorland argues that such programs promote "unhealthy sex absorption" and "primitive behavior."[15]

Further, "Dr. [Wanda] Franz has shown not only that comprehensive sex education goes contrary to adolescent cognitive development, but that it is also inappropriate relative to the state of adolescent moral development."[16] Melvin Anchell warns that all preteen sex instruction is risky. He points out that sex instruction, even to very young children, may include "repeated demonstrations of nudity, genital anatomy, and how humans and animals mate." Children as young as three to six years old may thus "become fixed in the need for exhibitionistic and voyeuristic pleasure" later in life. Further, many studies have shown that when children are permitted to watch people mate, "they may come to regard the sex act as a sadistic subjugation— an abuse—of the female."[17]

A large amount of psychoanalytic research suggests that most adult sexual offenders "are products of premature sexual seduction in early childhood" and may not be limited to actual molestation per se. This may extend to "overexposure to sexual activities, including sex courses in the classroom."[18]

Anchell notes that early childhood is not the only danger zone. The second sexual period, ages six to twelve, is known as latency. In this period children are most educable and a good deal of the child's moral development is at stake. Sex education here interferes with proper sexual development by keeping the sexual impulses aroused, "disrupting both sexual growth and personal and cultural achievements. Not infrequently, sex educators applaud the bold, immodest behavior of their student protégés and proclaim such behavior a sign of increased social acumen. In truth, the personality traits that they applaud are the early characteristics of the psychopath—that is, an individual who cares about others only insofar as they can serve some purpose for him."[19]

Harold wasn't a model student, but he did his best. Nor was he sexually promiscuous, at least until after his eighth grade class in sex education. Harold had a poor self-image and had suffered from his parents' divorce and other problems at home. His sex ed class encouraged him to think about how much fun sex was and about how much he needed someone to love and care for him. Harold thought that sex might be a good way to find love and affection.

But after two disastrous sexual encounters in the ninth grade, Harold became increasingly withdrawn. He also became more aggressive and antisocial. He began to express the idea that he could do whatever he wanted because, not only did no one care about him, but also his own teachers had told him there were no moral absolutes—so nothing was ultimately wrong.

After experimenting with drugs, Harold began selling them to other students. Again, Harold explained that he had been taught by his teachers that the values that were "right for him" were the values he should defend. In the end, what became "right for Harold" was unbridled drug and alcohol abuse, resentment of authority, and crimes such as "breaking and entering" and stealing cars. Finally, Harold set fire to the school, which earned him two years in the county jail.

Anchell observes that psychopathy in preteens has reached "alarming proportions. Preteen murders, pregnancy, and criminality are becoming more frequent." Yet he notes that the preteen who has not been sexually disturbed is typically a responsible individual and rarely involved in sociopathic behavior. "It is impossible to draw a straight line between crime statistics and pre-teen sexual indoctrination; but it is absurd to ignore the powerful psychosexual forces to which young people are being exposed."[20]

He points out that sex educators not only help students to distrust the values of their parents and Judeo-Christian religion, but they also encourage inexperienced youths to develop their own values, which often amounts to having few or no values at all. "An examination of any ordinary sex education 'teacher's guide and resource manual' makes the point. In this regard, the manuals provided to schools by Planned Parenthood are classic."[21]

Modern sex education assumes a new morality based on a false assumption—that teenagers can make wise decisions if given "proper," value-free information about sex and relationships. Consider the widely taught belief that living together in a "trial marriage" actually increases one's chances for a successful marriage. Kinsey researcher Wardell Pomeroy teaches, "For those planning to marry eventually, early intercourse can be a training ground. Valuable lessons can be learned by getting a taste of what it's like to live with someone else."[22] Thus, he claims, premarital intercourse among teenagers considering marriage "will be a big help in finding out if they're really compatible or not."[23]

But, despite widespread claims that living together prior to marriage is a healthful approach toward assessing compatibility, recent research reveals that just the opposite is true. "The assumption is that a 'trial marriage' will help to screen out incompatible couples, thereby producing future marriages with greater satisfaction, communication, and commitment. However, studies of cohabitors show that the opposite tends to occur."[24]

Perhaps we should have known all along that indoctrinating children in value-*free* sex education could not assist them in making *moral* decisions about sexuality. Regardless, preteens and adolescents cannot be expected to make the same kinds of rational decisions that adults do, just because they know more about sex. (Even adults often make poor choices morally.) Information about sex and making wise decisions concerning it are two different matters. The results of modern sex education have proven that, given a wide range of choices about sex and sexual lifestyles, teenagers will often choose what is *not* in their best interest.

Unfortunately, "morality" is almost a dirty word today. Parents who oppose the existing system and want to see sex education based upon legitimate moral standards have been labeled as "censors," "extremists," "fundamentalists," people denying academic freedom, returning to the dark ages, and being "anti-education." Unfortunately, when parents assumed that the professionals knew more than they did and surrendered their children's sex education, the end result has been the current situation.

To instruct teens and preteens in explicit sexuality, telling them that they really won't be able to control their sexual urges and will sooner or later be engaging in sexual behavior, all the while telling them that there are no moral absolutes and that they must decide what is "right for them," is not the way to avoid teenage promiscuity, pregnancy, or sexually transmitted diseases.

Anchell observes that the sex educators seem unable to understand the consequences of their own programs, which are, in part, responsible for the pregnancies, STDs, abortions, perversions, suicides, and psychological problems so common today. While these educators allege they are protecting young people "from the influence of sexually inhibited parents and outmoded religious teachings," it is these very teachings that offer the reconfirmation of normal sexual development. "Today's children and adolescents need an educational system that upholds the family and basic Judaeo-Christian morality—a morality that supports . . . and sustains civilized life, rather than undermining it."[25]

THE MYTHS OF SEX EDUCATION

In *The Myths of Sex Education* Josh McDowell discusses six false assumptions of sex educators. They are summarized below.

THE FIRST MYTH is that comprehensive sex education is value free and morally neutral.

It frequently promotes the permissive sexual values of those who have authored the programs and is anything *but* value free and morally neutral. It is far too sexually explicit. The homosexual and lesbian communities, and others who wish to promote sexual freedom, use these programs and are even involved in their curriculum instruction in order to more widely promote their own agenda to society by influencing our children (see chap. 10).

THE SECOND MYTH is that comprehensive sex education increases responsible teen contraception.

Setting up clinics and dispensing contraceptives in high schools and colleges only produces a climate of legitimacy for sexual activity. Far from decreasing sex, contraception programs assume the social acceptance of widespread sexual activity. That is why comprehensive sex education has dramatically increased teenage premarital sexual activity, abortions, STDs, and so on.

Douglas Kirby, the former research director for the Center for Population Options, an organization committed to comprehensive sex education in school-based health clinics, released the results of a multiyear study in 1988: "We have been engaged in a research project for several years on the impact of school based clinics. . . . We find basically that there is no measurable impact upon the use of birth control, nor upon pregnancy rates or birth rates."[26]

It is a social fact that increased availability of contraceptives brings increased sexual activity and all the problems associated with it. Promoting contraceptives to our teenagers will not reduce teen pregnancy, it will not reduce teen abortion, and it will certainly not reduce teen sexual activity, AIDS, and other STDs. Although sex education does lead to increased use of contraceptives, the result is negative, not positive. School-based contraception clinics and birth control education has resulted in tens of millions of teenagers pursuing sexual activity who might not otherwise have been able to legitimize their pursuits. In addition, teenagers frequently do not use contraceptives properly even after sound instruction.

THE THIRD MYTH is that comprehensive sex education does not increase teen promiscuity.

McDowell and others have shown that it does greatly increase teenage sexual promiscuity.[27] Even many educators and former supporters of contraception have themselves confessed that the availability of contraceptives has made teenagers (and the adult population as well) more, not less, permissive.[28]

If comprehensive sex education programs provide students with explicit technical instruction for having sex and then assure teenagers there are numerous benefits to premarital sex, can anyone seriously think this will *decrease* sexual activity? When humanist manifestos declare that each person has the right to determine his own sexual conduct, and when seminars given by comprehensive sex educators warn teenagers not to listen to their parents' advice, should we be surprised at the results?[29]

THE FOURTH MYTH is that comprehensive sex education reduces teenage pregnancies.

"Numerous studies reveal that family planning methods in comprehensive sex education produce a dramatic *increase* in teenage pregnancy."[30] Even Planned Parenthood confesses that school-based sex education is not reducing pregnancies. Dr. Debra Ann Dawson admits, "The final result to emerge from the [comprehensive national] analysis is that neither pregnancy education nor contraceptive education exerts any significant effect on the risk of premarital pregnancy among sexually active teenagers—a finding that calls into question the argument that formal sex education is an effective tool for reducing adolescent pregnancy."[31]

THE FIFTH MYTH is that comprehensive sex education reduces teen abortions.

This belief is based on an incorrect assumption that an increased use of contraceptive practices will reduce pregnancies and, therefore, abortions. But as many researchers have shown, the availability of contraceptives *increases* pregnancies. By definition it, therefore, also *increases* abortions. Both the dramatic increase in pregnancies from

1970 to 1980 (40 percent) and abortions (123 percent) are concurrent with the increase in the numbers of comprehensive sex education programs and the availability of contraceptives to teens.[32]

In our book *When Does Life Begin? And 39 Other Tough Questions About Abortion*, we show some of the terrible consequences of abortion. Any program that helps to increase abortion is doing a serious injustice to public health. In fact, McDowell presents figures to indicate the possibility that there have not been merely 30 million abortions since Roe v. Wade, but possibly as many as 170 million. As he comments, "If these figures are anywhere close to being true, no wonder the abortionists don't want us to know exactly how many abortions are taking place." [33]

THE SIXTH MYTH is that comprehensive sex education will succeed with greater funding.

Since these programs are not effective in any of their stated goals, pouring more money into them is simply throwing it away. Dramatically increasing the funding of these programs will only dramatically increase their failures.

In conclusion, so-called comprehensive sex education is part of the problem of the modern sexual tragedy—a major part. Until these programs are either thoroughly revised or abandoned, there will be no solution to the problems we face.

McDowell offers seven strategies for resolving the sexual crisis among teenagers: (1) including and involving parents; (2) teaching the consequences of promiscuity; (3) teaching moral values; (4) teaching abstinence; (5) eliminating mixed messages concerning abstinence; (6) implementing abstinence-based programs; and (7) using commercially available resources for abstinence education. We encourage readers to purchase this book and review these important materials, as well as Newman and Richards, *Healthy Sex Education in Your Schools*.[34]

Value-Free Sex Education—
Or Indoctrination in Permissiveness?

They're Teaching Our Kids What
They Don't Want to Know

*Having sex is a joyful and enriching experience at any age. It begins
when we're very young.*

Wardell B. Pomeroy

Comprehensive sex education has permitted a vocal minority of
so-called "value-free, morally neutral" sex educators, including
Planned Parenthood and others, to harm children's lives. Although
their motives are often well-intentioned, some sex educators are
hoping to indoctrinate young people with their own attitudes of sexual
"enlightenment." As McDowell states, "Perhaps the greatest deception perpetrated on the parents of teens in this country is the myth of
value-free, morally neutral sex education. I have never met anyone,
let alone a teacher, who can act as a neutral catalyst on any subject,
let alone sex. Whenever a kid is around an adult, the adult's values
will be communicated either verbally or nonverbally."[1] In other words,
adult teachers cannot help but communicate their own sexual values—
and in our nation today, these are frequently anti-Christian.

"VALUE FREE" IT'S NOT

We have been told that any teaching about sex in the public schools
should be entirely free of moral judgments. We must let children
decide for themselves what their behavior will be. But as former
Secretary of Education William Bennett points out, "it is a very odd
kind of teaching—very odd because it does not teach. . . . It displays
a conscious aversion to making moral distinctions. . . . The words of
morality, of a rational, mature morality, seem to have been banished

from this sort of sex education."[2]

Indeed, "moralistic education" is often ridiculed by these authorities and held up as sophomoric and destructive precisely *because* it seeks to influence children to accept a moral viewpoint. Thus, because it is a moral judgment to tell students that certain sexual activities are wrong, such instruction is said to be unacceptable. But is this being "value free"? Is this being morally neutral? Or is this seeking to influence others with relative or even antimoral values?

As former educator and psychology teacher Ann E. Morgan comments:

> Despite its claims of being "neutral," comprehensive sex-ed is not truly value free. Listing certain options gives value to them, with the endorsement of the authority of the State and the school behind those options. If, for example, a parent has taught his child that abortion is wrong, and the school [or State] says that it is not, but merely one of many options, this undermines the parent's attempt at inculcating that value.
>
> For years, liberals have used this as an argument against school prayer, saying that the very presence of prayer at school lends the credibility and authority of the school and State to that prayer; it would then possibly undermine what a parent was trying to teach—even if the child did not participate.[3]

Even W. R. Coulson, cofounder and research director of a project to test "affective," or value-free, education, finally recognized that this program, in effect, *encouraged* destructive behavior—and he said that he and others associated with value-free education owed the nation's parents an apology.

> The research is clear and consistent on this, with numerous studies yielding the same results: getting facilitation [value-free discussion of subjects] instead of teaching [morality] causes students to become more interested in making decisions than in doing what is right: right becomes whatever they decide. The bad effects don't end with smoking. Youthful experimentation with sex, alcohol, marijuana and a variety of other drugs—whatever is popular at the time—has been shown to follow affective, value-free education quite predictably; we now know that after these classes, students become more prone to give in to temptation than if they had never been enrolled.[4]

As Drs. Alexandra and Vernon Mark argue, "Most of the proponents of permissive sex education pride themselves on the fact that they do not make value judgments; they studiously avoid preaching. That is what they say. It might even be what they think. But that doesn't make it true. What they are doing is systematically and relentlessly imposing *their* value judgments on our society, and they are indeed preaching—their personal brand of sexual religion."[5]

Those who claim to teach our children moral neutrality and to champion value-free programs frequently demand that parents and churches not impose *their* morality, especially sexual abstinence, on their own children or other teenagers. In other words, the very ones who speak in the name of neutrality demand that (1) the moral views of parents be restricted or silenced and (2) their own amoral or immoral views be encouraged or imposed upon the nation's children. "How bold, how ludicrous, how moral oriented, how value oriented! I can't believe the gall of anyone insisting that parents encourage their own teens to turn against parental values in order to follow a view which is the exact opposite. Such a demand is anything but morally neutral."[6]

"INDOCTRINATION" IT IS

An example of indoctrination in permissiveness can be seen in two popular books—*Boys and Sex*, and *Girls and Sex*—by Wardell B. Pomeroy, coauthor of the famous Kinsey Reports. Pomeroy is well aware of the problems surrounding human sexuality.

> There is no universal activity engaged in by human beings that causes so much unhappiness, disappointment, and misery as what happens in people's sex lives. . . . I learned this for the first time a half century ago when I helped to compile what came to be known as the Kinsey Reports. During the research that produced these landmark books, I took the sexual histories of more than eight thousand different people (plus two thousand others in later years) ranging from young children to individuals over ninety. They came from every part of the United States and from every social and economic level; far too often I found that their sex lives had been a record of unhappiness, disappointment, even misery.[7]

He also wrote, "We're supersaturated with sex, and there's nothing new. But if that's so, why is it that the offices of sex therapists everywhere in the country are filled with people who are having all kinds of problems?"[8]

Further, Pomeroy is well aware of the destructive potential of teenage intercourse: "That teenage intercourse can also generate its own problems is evident in the high suicide rate among teens, where it's a factor in a surprising number of cases and adds to adolescent despair over the state of the world and their own lives."[9] But given conditions in the world today, is it really so surprising that teenage intercourse is a significant factor in the teen suicide rate?

Pomeroy is aware of these problems, but he still encourages teenagers to have sex as early as possible. He thinks these problems only result from a repressive puritanical, religious view toward sex. Thus, he is content that the old morality "has virtually disappeared" except for "remnants" in various parts of society, "notably those who follow strict religious beliefs" (e.g., that "early intercourse without the sanctity of marriage is morally wrong" and that women "were supposed to be pure and undefiled right up to the altar").[10]

Those such as Pomeroy do not understand (1 Corinthians 2:14) that sex is a gift from God that is properly subject to His loving commands. If God is the author of sex, then having sex in accordance with God's purposes will not only produce the best sex but also the best sexual development. To reject and violate God's commands about sex will produce the problems we see about us today because sexual permissiveness is destructive to the created order and hence ultimately self-destructive.

But Pomeroy believes that the real problem is ignorance about sex—even though the last two decades have educated children and adults in sexuality far surpassing that of any other generation. Even Pomeroy confesses, "Never in the history of our country have sexual customs and behavior changed so radically in so short a time, and never has there been so much public acceptance of human sexuality."[11]

But it is not ignorance of sex that is the problem. It is the active promotion of "animal" sexuality encouraged by influential men like Pomeroy. How do we know this? Because it is the biblical view of sex that is not only the safest by far but that also leads to greatest sexual contentment in marriage.

The Bible teaches that sex is a gift from God. It is something wonderful that is to be enjoyed, but reserved for marriage. Parents who have educated their children in biblical standards concerning sexuality—and children who have obeyed biblical injunctions— characteristically have few of the problems encountered by those who are educated in liberal attitudes toward sex. They do not have problems with guilt, emotional rejection from broken relationships, suicides, sexually transmitted diseases, unwanted pregnancies, abortion, or the other problems that accompany promiscuity.

Even though the back cover of *Boys and Sex* claims that Pomeroy's book "does not advocate permissiveness," that is not true. Pomeroy advocates permissiveness to such an extent that he encourages adolescents to have sexual intercourse. What is the age level that Pomeroy writes for? His intended audience is teens and preteens. "I think of girls who are no more than ten, eleven or twelve as part of my audience. You're already reading books written for your age group by such very popular writers as Judy Blume, containing quite explicit sexual situations."[12] He believes his view is the proper, enlightened, and "moral" view, and other views are inferior or wrong. He tells these ten-, eleven-, and twelve-year-old girls that sex is "the most natural thing in the world and the most common human activity. You and your friends have a sexual freedom today that no previous generation enjoyed."[13] He claims that young girls today understand that they are "far more likely" to make proper social and sexual adjustments in later life if they learn to be "warm, open, responsive, and sexually unafraid."[14] He emphasizes that "teenage sex should be a learning experience, not a frightening one."[15]

Condemning the fact that our society "still plays the mindless game of 'good girl' and 'bad girl',"[16] he encourages young girls to be sexually experimental and claims that teenage sex can improve their sex lives when they are finally married. Pomeroy argues (incorrectly), "The longer a girl delays experiencing [an orgasm], whatever the source, the more difficult it may be to have it later in life. . . . It's a demonstrable fact that girls who have orgasm when they are young— that is, up to fifteen—are those who experience the least difficulty having it later on. . . . Clearly, a girl who learns what orgasm is at an early point in her adolescence is going to have a more fulfilling time later on."[17]

In addition, childhood sex play among members of the opposite and *same* sex is held to be beneficial. "As I have said, a girl who has had sex play with girls and boys her own age is likely to have benefited from the experiences in one way or another, particularly her later adjustments to sex, and consequently they're valuable, even if some of them turned out badly."[18]

On the other hand, the girl who decides to remain a virgin until she is married is told that is probably a mistake. "For those planning to marry eventually, early intercourse can be a training ground. Valuable lessons can be learned by getting a taste of what it's like to live with someone else. . . . After marriage, many girls regret that they didn't have premarital intercourse because they now realize what a long, slow learning process it can be."[19]

Pomeroy confesses that the very morality he attempts to undermine is what prevented most girls from engaging in more premarital intercourse—hence his opposition to it. "As many as 80 percent of girls say the reason they didn't have more intercourse before marriage was because of strong moral objections that prevented them."[20]

Nor does Pomeroy have a problem with lesbianism. "Finally, I want to emphasize that homosexual [i.e., lesbian] relationships can be as pleasurable, as deep, and as worthwhile as heterosexual ones, even though society still has strong feelings against them."[21]

In *Boys and Sex* he goes even further. He tells young boys, "Everyone is entitled to a rewarding sex life. . . . We have learned in this century that having sex is a joyful and enriching experience *at any age*. It begins when we are *very young*."[22] He hopes his advice "will dispel any guilt or fear about sexual behavior they may have."[23]

And he puts parents in what he thinks is their proper place: "Parents need to get off their moral soapboxes and speak casually about sex. . . . Everyone knows the official attitude, which is expressed in codes and laws. . . . Those who hold to the official attitude are intolerant of any kind of sexual behavior they believe isn't 'normal.' They measure normality by what *they* do or think they should do."[24]

But such an attitude is only an illustration of the hypocrisy of many sexologists who reject all moral absolutes but one—*their* absolute right to indoctrinate young children with their own sexual agenda. Yet Pomeroy has the gall to explain to parents that he is not advocating sexual permissiveness. "I hope parents will accept the idea that I am being neither permissive nor strict. I am not urging boys to engage in sexual behavior of any kind. A great majority of them, with only an insignificant percentage of exceptions, have already engaged and are engaging in some kind of sexual behavior, and once started, they aren't likely to stop. . . . Simply telling children to stop sexual activity, which fills them with guilt and fear in the process or makes them feel ridiculous, is the kind of approach that is certain to fail."[25]

Pomeroy goes on to explain the "good news." The good news is that "there appears to be a growing number of people who don't view sex in such absolute [moral] terms. . . . The more liberal of these people think it ought to be possible for young people to have relatively complete sexual freedom. . . . [They say] the healthiest attitude about sex is to regard it as fun, and the more of it a person has, the better off he will be, psychologically and physically."[26] What Pomeroy believes is that "sex in *all its forms* is a normal, natural part of being human."[27] If such an attitude isn't permissive, what is?

Pomeroy also argues—wrongly and in biased fashion—that abstinence is impossible for preteens and teenagers. "Those who still think that [sex is] something boys and girls can just postpone until they're in their twenties don't understand human sexuality."[28] He informs young boys, "Eventually, as you start to grow up, you'll be having sexual encounters of one kind or another."[29] Here, Pomeroy has superimposed his own liberal view of sex upon the behavior of young boys he knows nothing about.

Continuing to reflect Kinseyan philosophy, he argues, "We're all mammals, and so our sexual behavior, which is like that of other mammals, is natural. Other mammals of the nonhuman kind engage in nearly every kind of sexual activity that we do. So from that standpoint, there's really nothing humans do sexually that's abnormal."[30] (This response was given, in part, to answer a question, "What is abnormal sex?")

Although he claims he does not encourage boys to engage in homosexual behavior, he says this:

> With the greater sexual freedom we enjoy today, permitting more experimentation, some people have discovered they enjoy relations with both sexes. In doing this, they are only following what we learn as children. Sexually, children act very much like other mammals. All religions believe that what separates men and women from their fellow mammals is their souls, and that is a matter of faith. But massive scientific evidence also shows many similarities in sexual behavior between people and animals. . . . All species of mammals have homosexual relations. . . . Since we are all mammals, then, it is reasonable to wonder why all boys don't engage in homosexual behavior. They don't, of course, and I'm not suggesting they should.[31]

But he goes on to observe that the basic reason boys should give serious consideration to whether or not they want to engage in homosexual behavior is largely because of the conflicts about homosexuality in society, not because homosexuality is wrong. It just means a person may end up with more problems. "Homosexuality is much more a state of mind than it is actual behavior. It's simply a matter of sexual preference."[32]

As he did for young girls, Pomeroy encourages young boys to engage in early premarital sex and intercourse: "Boys who start having sex the earliest—sex of some kind, that is—are the ones most likely to have the longest active sex lives and to have the most sex when they are older."[33]

> If you're having sex with someone you have no intention of marrying or living with, it can be a good training ground for a more committed experience later on. . . . For the adolescent boy and girl who start intercourse with the idea that they will get married later on, it will be a big help in finding out if they're really compatible or not. . . . It's like taking a car out on a test run before you buy it. . . . For a really satisfactory sexual relationship, techniques have to be learned, and that is where early intercourse can be a help in later life. It is easier to learn when we are young."[34]

But why wouldn't it be better to learn about sexual techniques with someone you love in a permanent marriage relationship offering maturity, security, and stability?

After giving boys "several good reasons for having intercourse,"[35] Pomeroy talks about some of the consequences, such as pregnancy and STDs. But the damage has already been done. Young boys and girls have been told that at their age sex is good and normal and to be expected. They only need proper education about sex to enjoy sexually fulfilling lives at any age.

The problem with this view is that it is simply unworkable, not to mention destructive—psychologically, morally, and spiritually. That is what teenagers have been doing for twenty years, and look at the results. Pomeroy thinks ignorance is still the problem even when we are no longer ignorant. But the real problem is permissiveness.

If you were a parent, how would you like your ten- or eleven-year-old son or daughter to read the following? "A boy may put his mouth on the girl's vagina, or she may put hers on his penis, or they may do this at the same time. That usually is leading up to intercourse. . . . If you haven't begun to do any of these things yet, you may be wondering, 'Why do people do this, anyway?' There are three good reasons. The most obvious is that it's so much fun."[36] Pomeroy also gives specific masturbation instructions,[37] specific instruction on condom use, intercourse itself, and various sexual positions.[38] Remember, this is all intended for young *boys,* not adults. (*Straight Talk,* by Marilyn Ratner and Susan Chamlim, is another sex manual used by Planned Parenthood. It also refers to masturbation when it says, "It's perfectly OK, however, for a parent to help an older child, say four and older, to find a private place for this activity.")[39]

According to Pomeroy, fantasy during masturbation involving incest, group sex, and rape are not generally to be considered harmful.

> [Boys] might have fantasies of having sex with their sisters, a teacher, or even their mothers or fathers. Sometimes they imagine an orgy in which several boys and girls, or just boys, are taking part. At other times, it's having sex with a particular boy or girl, or even a grown man or woman. They may think about forcing themselves to have sex with them, or being forced themselves. These daydreams needn't be (and usually aren't) any more harmful than the common daydreams boys have about being the best baseball player in the world or becoming a millionaire.[40]

We question whether such daydreams are really harmless. What we are inwardly is what we become outwardly. One can only wonder how many convicted sex offenders' amoral fantasy lives may have led to greater and greater excesses and finally criminal behavior. If what Pomeroy says is true, then why should anyone consider it a problem to encourage even worse sexual fantasies? Or, why restrict yourself to fantasy? If there are no moral absolutes and any given sex behavior is "right" for you and someone else, why restrict anything?

For example, although acknowledging necrophilia (sex with a dead person) as being considered immoral by almost everyone, he classifies bestiality (sex with an animal) as "a somewhat different matter." He notices that it is "practiced around the world and has been known as far back as the ancient world. In our time, about 4 percent of city boys and 17 percent of farm boys, according to Kinsey's figures, engaged in sexual behavior with animals, and 4 percent of both city and farm girls had done it. As to whether it is immoral or not, that depends entirely on the point of view."[41]

In response to the question, "What would happen if a boy had intercourse with an animal?" he encourages boys that have had this experience to not feel bad about it: "You would be best advised to keep any knowledge of it to yourself so you can avoid either ridicule or punishment, or both. You can feel secure in your knowledge that you're not a monster, no matter what society may think about it."[42]

Pomeroy may think he isn't preaching, but he is. What's worse is that this moral "neutrality" is often limited to sex alone. Never do the value-free educators teach a morally neutral approach to cheating, violence, rape, stealing, lying, or drug use. "Just imagine if a teacher, in a unit on alcohol, were to describe in full detail the methods of getting drunk, or spend time talking about drunk driving without offering any moral judgment as to whether driving while intoxicated was right or wrong, but says, 'If you decide to drive and drink, here are some ways to avoid detection: this is 85 percent safe, this one 92 percent.' We would think the teacher incompetent."[43] But when the exact same thing is done in the area of teen sexuality, we somehow think the teacher is "enlightened" and really serving the interests of our children.

Further, such sex "education" fails to recognize the almost universal immaturity of teenage decision making. When they are exposed to a variety of "equally moral choices," teenagers easily become confused or give up. What else should we expect? What teenagers need is consistent, firm moral standards to be upheld by those in authority—not a permissiveness that may destroy them.

When we teach our own children to be value free and morally neutral in their sexuality, is it surprising that they become adults who are not honest when society or their sexual partners ask them whether they have AIDS or other STDs? If we denigrate morality in elementary school, junior high, and high school, why should we expect adults who are a product of such education to all of a sudden adopt moral values in their relations with others?

Finally, many comprehensive sex education programs open the door for extreme explicitness in sexual instructional materials. Comprehensive sex education may teach children things like "sexual sickeys grow up in homes in which sex is taboo." And, "parents who quote Scriptures against homosexuality are 'irrational'; their minds are perverted."[44]

Would an individual committed to moral neutrality include the following in children's sex-education instruction?

- "If you feel your parents are overprotective, their message   may not be helpful. If they seem to fear your sexuality, or if they don't want you to be sexual at all until some distant time, you may feel you have tuned out their voice entirely. Or it may be strong enough only to make you feel guilty. But if your parents seem to trust your judgment and basically just want you to take care of yourself, their voice of carefulness can help you make decisions you will be glad about."[45] Is such advice neutral? Is it without values?
- Discussions of a child's "coming out" as a homosexual.
- Instruction concerning gay and bi-sexual teenagers who "need to meet other people like them for friendship and support."
- "Gay bars often are among the only places to find openly gay people. Many teens find their way into gay bars despite being under the drinking age. Bars have been a lifeline for lesbian and gay people."
- Specific instructions on lesbians' sexual techniques.
- Specific instructions on male homosexual techniques.
- Encouragement for teenagers to seek out prostitutes, "Do you want a convenient warm body? Buy one. That's right. There are women who have freely chosen the business. Buy one."[46]

Some sex educators' workshops teach that "children from the sixth grade on must come to accept [homosexuality] as normal." They even offer children "workshops" where they role-play homosexual and lesbian relationships. Some districts even refuse to permit students to pass their "health" class without first buying condoms.[47]

The CDC pamphlet "Teens and AIDS" offers the following advice:

THE TEENAGER'S BILL OF RIGHTS. . . .

I have the right to decide whether to have sex and who to have it with. . . . I have the right to buy and use con-doms. . . . Use a latex condom for *any* sex where the penis enters another person's body. That means vaginal sex (penis into a woman's vagina), oral sex (penis into the mouth), and anal sex (penis into the butt). . . . Guys can get used to the feel of condoms while masturbating.[48]

Pamphlets published by the Gay Men's Health Crisis and distributed at some high schools are so pornographic they cannot even be described publicly (e.g., "Safer Sex Guidelines for Gay Men" distributed at Martin Luther King High School, NYC).

The above are only some examples of "morally neutral" sex education. They are cited in various books and pamphlets used or published by Planned Parenthood, including *Changing Bodies, Changing Lives; The New Our Bodies, Ourselves; Boys and Sex; Girls and Sex; One Teenager in Ten: Writings by Gay and Lesbian Youth;* and *Straight Talk: Sexuality Education for Parents and Kids 4–7.*

There is little doubt that teenage promiscuity today is largely the result of the morally "neutral" sexual education in our junior and senior high schools and the carefree attitude toward sexuality in modern culture. McDowell is right when he says, "I firmly believe that value-free, morally neutral sex education is largely responsible for the sobering statistics on rape in our country."[49]

How Safe Is Abortion?*
Physical and Psychological Risks

One teenager recalls the following: "I had an abortion today. I had an abortion, and I have been sick, physically sick, ever since. But the vomiting and the cramps cannot compare with how I feel mentally and emotionally at this moment. I know that abortion is wrong. So, you wonder why I did it? Because I was stuck, that's why. I got myself into a situation that I saw no other way out of. How did I get myself into this situation? I don't really know."[1]

The physically and emotionally damaging consequences of the STD epidemic are not the only results of the sexual revolution. Another is as frequently overlooked as it is underreported: the personal consequences of abortion.

In the last twenty or thirty years some thirty to forty million abortions have been performed in America. Women were promised that these procedures were safe. In this chapter we will show why that claim is not true. Further information on abortion is available in *When Does Life Begin? And 39 Other Tough Questions About Abortion*. (The Conservative Book Club labeled this book the "best pro-life manual available anywhere.")[2]

Most people continue to believe that abortion is a safe procedure— at least for the mother. Those who support abortion in this country constantly inform us that there is nothing to be concerned about. "In comprehensive sex education, abortion is viewed as an integral subject, and it is often described as a perfectly safe procedure."[3] For

---

* The following material was excerpted from the authors' book *When Does Life Begin? and 39 Other Tough Questions About Abortion* (Dallas, Tex.: Word, 1990). Used by permission.

example, Dr. Jane Hodgson of the University of Minnesota is emphatic that "[this] is something we ought to be honest about. Abortion is a very safe procedure. There is no question about it being safe. Dr. Koop documented this after months and months of research."[4]

But not only is Hodgson wrong on abortion safety, she has misrepresented C. Everett Koop. According to many published interviews, Koop believes that abortion not only carries certain physical risks but also believes that, eventually, serious psychological effects will be proven. In essence, all Koop stated in his famous "report" on the psychological complications of abortion (a three-page letter) was that the current studies are flawed because they do not examine the problem of psychological consequences for a long enough period.[5]

Compare the above statement by Hodgson assuring women that abortion is medically safe with the following from an official research paper presented to the former U.S. Surgeon General: "While there are a number of studies with contradictory findings with respect to the medical outcomes of abortion, the following risks have been identified: tubal infertility, subsequent fetal malformations, cervical trauma, ectopic pregnancy, PID [Pelvic Inflammatory Disease], hemorrhaging, infertility, subsequent miscarriages, and death (Cates et al., 1983, Grimes, 1983, Harlap and Davies, 1975, Frank et al., 1985, Buehler et al., 1986)."[6]

After examining "the vast body of the world's medical literature on the subject," Thomas W. Hilgers, M.D., concluded, "The medical hazards of legally induced abortion are very significant and should be conscientiously weighed."[7]

PHYSICAL RISKS

Hundreds of thousands of women have already paid a physical price and many have paid the ultimate price for their abortion: thousands have died.[8]

Here is a brief *verbatim* list of the possible physical consequences that can come to those having abortions:

- Death
- Perforation of the uterus
- Bleeding requiring transfusion (with possible hepatitis or AIDS infection)
- Tearing of the cervix, with unknown impact upon cervical competence during subsequent pregnancies

- Anesthesia-related accidents, including convulsions, shock, and cardiac arrest from toxic reaction to the anesthetic used
- Pelvic inflammatory disease and possible associated infertility
- Unintended surgery, including laparotomy, hysterotomy, and hysterectomy
- Bladder perforation
- Bowel perforation
- Persistent bleeding
- Tissue retention
- Anemia
- Peritonitis (a serious infection of the membranous coat lining the abdominal cavity)
- Minor infections and fever of unknown origin
- Undetected tubal pregnancy
- Pulmonary emboli (obstruction of the pulmonary artery)
- Venous thrombophlebitis (inflammation of a vein developing before a blood clot)
- Depression
- Psychosis
- Suicide[9]

Many women who have experienced such problems are rightfully angry over never having been warned of such consequences prior to the abortion. The unfortunate fact is that none of these consequences can be predicted in advance. The woman who has an abortion is playing Russian roulette not only with her body but also with her ability to conceive in the future, with her own mental health, and even with the health of future children.[10]

Susan and Jim had been married for five years and had one child. Although they wanted another, they were simply not prepared for Susan's pregnancy. After agonizing reflection, they decided that Susan would have an abortion. The abortion procedure went well, but several days later complications began to develop. Susan began to have a high fever, severe stomach cramps, and swollen glands. Upon admission to the hospital, it was discovered that she had developed an infection of her reproductive organs as a direct result of her abortion. The result was permanent infertility.

Not only could Susan never have the second child she wanted, but her young son, when he found out about the abortion, became depressed and afraid for no apparent reason. Only after months of counseling did Susan and her husband discover that their son had harbored a secret fear that if "mommy and daddy" would take away his little brother or sister, they might "take him away" too.

Here are some official health statistics that reveal the dangers attached to having an abortion:

> Studies show that 20% to 30% of all suction and D and C abortions performed in hospitals will result in long term, negative side effects relating primarily to fertility and reproduction.[11]

> Every type of abortion procedure carries significant risks. . . . Overall, the rate of immediate and short term complications is no less than 10%. . . . The evidence indicates that the actual morbidity rate is probably much higher.[12]

> The technique of saline abortion was originally developed in the concentration camps of Nazi Germany. In Japan, where abortion has been legalized since the 1940s, the saline abortion technique has been outlawed because it is "extremely dangerous." Indeed, in the United States saline abortion is second only to heart transplants as the elective surgery with the highest fatality rate. Despite this fact, state laws attempting to prohibit saline abortions because of their great risks to aborting women have been declared unconstitutional by the courts.[13]

> Frequent complications associated with prostaglandin abortions include spontaneous ruptures in the uterine wall, convulsions, hemorrhage, coagulation defects, and cervical injury. Incomplete abortions are also very common.[14] A high risk of infection is common to all forms of abortion. . . . Many infections are dangerous and life-threatening, and severe pain will typically prompt the patient to seek emergency treatment. But [even though] the majority of infections are of a milder order . . . long term damage may still result.[15]

> Studies have shown that a woman's risk of an ectopic pregnancy dramatically increases following an abortion. . . . Treatment of an ectopic pregnancy requires major surgery. . . . [In addition] according to one study, the risk of a second trimester miscarriage increases tenfold following a vaginal abortion.[16]

Reminiscent of cases of criminal negligence, these women were never informed of abortion risks or were assured that it was an entirely safe procedure. That the image of *safety* is vital to the abortion industry is obvious—that the falseness of this image is deliberately hidden is inexcusable.

> The reported immediate complication rate, alone, of abortion is no less than 10%. In addition, studies of long-range complications show rates no less than 17% and frequently report complication rates in the range of 25 to 40%. One public hospital has even reported an overall complication rate following abortion of 70%!
>
> The extraordinary degree to which this evidence has been suppressed and ignored is shocking but instructive. . . .
>
> Indeed, the Supreme Court has given abortionists "super rights" which allow them to use any abortion technique they desire, no matter how dan-

gerous it may be, and the Court has made abortion clinics immune from any requirements for minimal standards of counseling.

According to this latter "constitutional right," abortion clinics are allowed, and even encouraged, not to tell their clients any of the risks associated with abortion. Instead, patients are to be kept in ignorance and thereby "protected" from "unnecessary fears" which may lead them to reevaluate the desirability of the abortion option.

The Court guarantees "freedom of choice" but denies the right to "informed choice." *Abortionists can legally withhold information* or even avoid their clients' direct questions, in order to ensure that the patient will agree to an abortion which will be, they assume, "in her best interests.". . .

Why is there such widespread silence about the dangers of legal abortion? Wasn't abortion legalized in order to *improve* health care for women rather than to encourage them to take unnecessary risks?[17]

Even the abortion-induced death rates are in all probability underreported and should be of much greater concern. Although the survey described below deals with information from 1968–1974, which mostly precedes Roe v. Wade, it is all the more relevant in light of the dramatic increase in the number of abortions.

As with other abortion complications, there is no accurate mechanism for gathering statistics about abortion-related deaths. The Supreme Court's abortion cases have struck down all requirements for reporting abortion-related complications and deaths on the grounds that such reporting might discourage women from seeking abortions. This new freedom allows abortionists and others to disguise abortion deaths under other categories when filling out death certificates. . . .

The degree to which abortion deaths are underreported is hinted at in the results of a 1974 survey which asked 486 obstetricians about their experience with complications resulting from legal abortions. . . . Extrapolation of this 6% sample rate to all 21,700 obstetricians in the U.S. in 1974 would indicate a probability of 1,300 patient deaths due to abortion-related complications during the six-year period between 1968 and 1974. But the actual number of deaths from legal abortions reported for that period was 52, only 5% of the projected figure. . . . Finally, this projection of 1,300 deaths between 1968 and 1974 is based on a survey of obstetricians only. Aborted women who died under the care of general practitioners or other health professionals would not be included in this survey, so the actual mortality rate, and cover-up, could be even worse.

What should be clear is that there is a major flaw in the mortality statistics for legal abortion. It is quite possible that only 5% to 10% of all deaths resulting from legal abortion are being reported as abortion-related. Even if 50% were being accurately reported, that extra margin of risk is far greater than women are being led to believe. Indeed, based on the reported abortion deaths alone, abortion is already the fifth leading cause of maternal death in the United States.

The most common causes of death from legal abortion include: hemorrhage, infection, blood clots in the lungs, heart failure, and anesthetic complications. These can occur after any type of abortion procedure and are generally unpredictable. . . . More frequently the death occurs after the patient leaves the clinic. . . .

Furthermore, it should be noted that abortion actually increases the chance of maternal death in later pregnancies.[18]

Subsequent injuries may not be reported for many reasons: the women who attempt this are ignored or turned away; they previously signed "consent" forms relieving the physician of responsibility for complications (these, however, are not legally binding); most abortions are personal or family secrets, so many women remain silent about complications and suffer in silence; sensitive gynecologists may not inform a woman that her problem is abortion related; finally, it is the abortionists who keep and control the statistics and have numerous motives for not reporting complications, whether immediate or long term.[19] The abortion industry is the largest unregulated industry in the nation; accountability is therefore minimized.[20]

What is clear from all this is that no physician in good conscience should perform an abortion: "Given the great psychological and physical risks posed by abortion, it is clear that the responsible physician, when interested in his client's overall health, would be extremely reluctant ever to recommend or perform an abortion."[21]

The abortion industry has everything to gain and nothing to lose by withholding data concerning the physical consequences of abortion. To report such information would be like someone's turning himself in to the IRS for an audit of last year's taxes and starting out the conversation by revealing a $100,000 bonus that he forgot to mention.

PSYCHOLOGICAL CONSEQUENCES

Melissa had fallen in love with a man she knew was probably not good for her. But she entered the relationship anyway and before long became pregnant. Her lover demanded that she get an abortion if she wanted to continue to see him. Melissa did this—not once, but three times. The result was permanent sterility and a brush with death. Today, even ten years later, Melissa still has a preoccupation with the babies she lost, flashbacks of her abortion experiences, depression, nightmares, and even "visitations" from the aborted children. Tragically, these kinds of experiences are variously reported among one-third to two-thirds of women who have had an abortion.[22]

The Royal College of Obstetricians and Gynecologists, in a survey of available psychiatric and psychological studies, found that serious psychological problems developed in many women after their abortions. The Royal College reported, "The incidence of serious, permanent psychiatric aftermath is variously reported as between 9 and 59%."[23]

As noted earlier, Dr. Koop never stated that abortions were psychologically safe. Due to media misreporting, that is how the nation has interpreted him, but falsely so.[24] In fact, Koop predicted that proper studies in the future will conclusively prove, scientifically and statistically, what he knows personally as a physician—that abortions are dangerous to a woman's mental health.[25]

Not everyone agrees that Koop is correct in his assessment that we must wait for future studies to prove that abortions do harm. Others believe the data are already sufficient to establish psychological dangers to abortion.[26] Even Koop was concerned enough to admit: "Ever since I've been at this job [Surgeon General] I have been trying to get CDC [Centers for Disease Control] to switch from studying the [abortion] mortality [deaths] to studying the morbidity [physical and psychological complications] which is what this [issue of the 'report'] is all about."[27]

Even Washington psychiatrist-obstetrician Julius Fogel, a doctor who performs abortions, admitted in 1971 before the Supreme Court decision: "I think every woman . . . has a trauma at destroying a pregnancy. . . . She is destroying herself. . . . A psychological price is paid. . . . It may be alienation, it may be a pushing away from human warmth, perhaps a hardening of the maternal instinct. Something happens on the deepest levels of a woman's consciousness when she destroys a pregnancy. I know that as a psychiatrist."[28]

In a 1989 interview (by this time he had performed some twenty thousand abortions), he noted, "There is no question about the emotional grief and mourning following an abortion. . . . Many come in [to the office even years later]—some are just mute, some hostile. Some burst out crying. . . . There is no question in my mind we are disturbing a life process."[29] What is becoming more and more evident is that, whether or not there are *immediate* psychological conse quences, they may emerge five, ten, fifteen, even twenty or thirty years later.

David Reardon, Ph.D., a contemporary scholar who has thoroughly researched the subject of abortion, agrees:

> A woman that a six-month post-abortion survey declares "well-adjusted" may experience severe trauma on the anniversary of the abortion date, or even many years later. This fact is attested to in psychiatric textbooks which affirm that: "The significance of abortions may not be revealed until later periods of emotional depression. During depressions occurring in the fifth or six decades of the patient's life, the psychiatrist frequently hears expressions of remorse and guilt concerning abortions that occurred twenty or more years earlier." In one study, the number of women who expressed "serious self-reproach" increased fivefold over the period of time covered by the study. . . .
>
> If and when the woman learns that the miscarriage may have been due to a previous abortion, the guilt and anguish can be overwhelming. In this sense, physical complications from abortion often contribute to psychological sequelae as well.
>
> On an even longer time scale, it has been observed that latent anxieties over a previous abortion frequently surface only with the onset of menopause.[30]

Joanne had never even considered the possibility of abortion until she found herself with an unwanted pregnancy, unmarried, and without a job. At the time, it seemed the only thing to do. But since that time, Joanne has suffered psychologically in ways that she would not have dreamed possible.

She was promised by her family physician and the abortionist that this was a safe procedure and that there would be no aftereffects. She discovered they were wrong. Within two years Joanne attempted suicide twice and after fifteen years suffered a relapse. She remains under psychiatric care.

The entire phenomenon of psychological aftereffects that takes place following abortions is known as "postabortion syndrome."[31] Early studies assumed that this syndrome would surface within a few months after the abortion—but it appears that with the majority of women it can be anywhere from five to thirty-five years later. Since abortion has been legalized in this country only since 1973, of course, no one can "scientifically, statistically" prove harmful long-term effects. But the data currently being gathered are more and more pointing to the devastating effects of postabortion syndrome.

Concerning the psychological complications of abortion, certain facts should be noted:

- For many reasons psychological complications are more difficult to scientifically prove than physical ones.
- Psychological complications are no less painful than physical ones; they may be more painful.
- The same obstructionism and underreporting found in the area of physical dangers are found here.[32] Abortion providers keep few, if any, records and have vested interests in maintaining the "abortion is safe" myth.
- The studies of abortion advocates are often biased.[33] Studies are usually short term and therefore incapable of revealing long-term effects. Immediate short-term studies (several weeks after) reveal lower rates of emotional problems primarily due to the *temporary* relief afforded by the cessation of the pregnancy, or a disorder known as "emotional paralysis."[34]

David Reardon offers a brief survey of the possible psychological complications due to abortion:

> A European study reported negative psychiatric manifestations following legal abortions in 55% of the women examined by psychiatrists.
>
> In the *American Journal of Psychiatry*, researchers reported that of 500 aborted women studied, 43% showed immediate negative responses. At the time of a later review, approximately 50% expressed negative feelings, and up to 10% of the women were classified as having developed "serious psychiatric complications."
>
> In one of the most detailed studies of post-abortion sequelae: "Anxiety, which if present after an abortion is felt very keenly, was reported by 43.1%. . . . Depression, one of the emotions likely to be felt with more than a moderate strength, was reported by 31.9% of women surveyed . . . 26.4% felt guilt, . . . [and] 18.1% felt no relief or just a bit. They were overwhelmed by negative feelings. Even those women who were strongly supportive of the right to abort reacted to their own abortions with regret, anger, embarrassment, fear of disapproval and even shame."
>
> In another paper, the same group of psychiatrists reported that when detailed interviews were performed, every aborted woman, "without exception" experienced "feelings of guilt or profound regret. . . . All the women felt that they had lost an important part of themselves."
>
> Another study of aborted women observed that 23% suffered "severe guilt." . . . One doctor reports: "Since abortion was legalized I have seen hundreds of patients who have had the operation. Approximately 10% expressed very little or no concern. . . ." Among the other 90% there were

all shades of distress, anxiety, heartache and remorse.[35]

Abortion cannot help but produce feelings of guilt and depression in most women. But in some women this increases the risk of suicide.

> Feelings of rejection, low self-esteem, guilt and depression are all ingredients for suicide, and the rate of suicide attempts among aborted women is phenomenally high. According to one study, women who have had abortions are nine times more likely to attempt suicide than women in the general population. The fact of high suicide rates among aborted women is well known among professionals who counsel suicidal persons. . . . There has been a dramatic rise in the suicide rate since the early 1970s when abortion was first legalized. Between 1978 and 1981 alone, the suicide rate among teenagers increased 500 percent.[36]

However, even those who suppress their feelings may be at risk:

> Suppressed feelings of remorse over abortion cause some women to suffer from psychosomatic illness. One study found that self-induced diseases among aborted women included abdominal discomfort, vomiting, pruritis vulvae, dysmenorrhea, frigidity, headaches, insomnia, fatigue, and ulcers. . . . Abortion has also been identified as the cause of psychotic and schizophrenic reactions. Symptoms frequently include extreme anxiety and feelings of paranoia.[37]

Although most abortion peddlers promise us that it is the *women* they are most concerned about, it is the women they also may help to destroy. Reardon's research reveals the following:

> Very few women can approach abortion without qualms or walk away from it without regrets. It is this ambivalence towards abortion, to use Francke's title term, which is the gateway to postabortion sequelae. For most women, abortion is not just an assault on their womb; it is an assault on their psyche. As we have seen, some women are literally forced into abortion by lovers, families, friends, or even by their physicians. Others slip into the abortion decision, restraining their doubts and questions, simply because it is the most visible and presumably the "easiest" way out of their dilemma. For these women, pro-abortion cliches replace investigation; blind trust supplants foresight. They assume abortion is safe because that is what they are told, and that is what they want to believe. They naively hope that they will have the strength to deal with the aftermath of abortion—even though they are choosing abortion because they feel they lack the strength to handle an unplanned pregnancy.
>
> Unfortunately, abortion does not build psychic strength; it drains it. . . . The abortion mentality, the institutional system of birth control counselors, abortionists, and clinics—all contribute to this faulty decision-making. As we will see later, abortion counselors are cosmetic figures who only reinforce the abortion choice, acting to support the woman's decision against the rebellion of her instinctive fears against such an unnatural procedure. Rather than urging the woman to confront her decision, reconsider it, and be prepared for its consequences, the counselors work to maintain the "safe

and easy" myth and encourage the woman to believe in abortion's tempting
lie: "Soon it will all be over."[38]

Anyone who has examined only a few dozen of the three hundred
studies conducted on the psychological aftermath of abortion cannot
doubt that abortions cause psychological problems to women.[39] What
is difficult to believe is the irresponsibility of those who claim it has
been "proven" that there are no psychological dangers.

If so, why are there now tens of thousands of women in groups such
as American Victims of Abortion (AVA), Victims of Choice, Women
Exploited By Abortion (WEBA), Post Abortion Counseling and Education (PACE), Healing Visions Network, and others? Why do hundreds of health care workers attend annual conferences at the
University of Notre Dame on postabortion counseling when there is
really no need?[40]

On March 16, 1989, Congress itself heard testimony of the psychological dangers of abortion from psychologist Wanda Franz, Ph.D., in
a special hearing on the medical and psychological impact of abortion:[41] "'Women who report negative after-effects from abortion know
exactly what their problem is. . . . They report horrible nightmares
of children calling to them from trash cans, of body parts, and blood.
When they are reminded of the abortion,' she continued, 'the women
re-experienced it with terrible psychological pain. . . . They feel
worthless and victimized because they failed at the most natural of
human activities—the role of being a mother.'"[42]

Other studies, such as the *Report on the Psychological Aftermath of
Abortion*[43] released in 1987, concluded: "The issue of reporting bias
is a very real concern in the examination of post abortion psychological
sequelae. . . . There is clear evidence of negative emotional aftermath
to abortion from the research results of existing investigations. This
is so in spite of either investigator or reporting bias." And, "It is the
conclusion of this report that negative psychological after-effects of
abortion exist and that they exist on a continuum from mild to severe,
and can be the basis of a diagnosed disorder identified as Post
Abortion Syndrome."[44]

The list of psychological abreactions [later responses] to induced abortion
is lengthy. . . : guilt, depression, grief, anxiety, sadness, shame, helplessness
and hopelessness, lowered self-esteem, distrust, hostility toward self and
others, regret, sleep disorders, recurring dreams, nightmares, anniversary

reactions, psychophysiological symptoms, suicidal ideation and behavior, alcohol and/or chemical dependencies, sexual dysfunction, insecurity, numbness, painful re-experiencing of the abortion, relationship disruption, communication impairment and/or restriction, isolation, fetal fantasies, self-condemnation, flashbacks, uncontrollable weeping, eating disorders, preoccupation, confused and/or distorted thinking, bitterness, and a sense of loss and emptiness."[45]

Further, this report cited several of the same problems found in other reports concerning the reluctance of women to report serious problems:

> The post-abortive woman's desire to keep her abortion experience a secret may prevent her from returning to the abortion provider or allowing follow-up to occur. Zimmerman (1977) found that the majority of women viewed abortion as a deviant act, one that they wished to keep a secret. Speckhard (1986) reported similar findings. Of the women she interviewed, 89 percent feared that others would learn of the abortion. . . . In addition, the post-abortive woman may . . . harbor very ambivalent, if not very negative feelings in regard to their abortion providers following the abortion experience (Lodl et al., 1985 and Joy, 1985). Thus, fears of "being found out," coupled with ambivalent feelings toward the abortion provider, often result in those women who are most distressed by their abortions being the most unlikely to return to the provider for follow-up. . . . The delayed onset of many of the symptoms of post abortion stress may cause confusion within the woman in this regard (i.e., as to the origin of her symptoms).
>
> Lastly, there are conflicting interests on the part of the abortion provider which may at times interfere with the provider's willingness to voluntarily furnish the government with evidences of post abortion morbidity. When morbidity data is collected, a well-intentioned provider may be reluctant to furnish this information because of an inherent conflict of interest.
>
> Thus it appears that although the federal government does obtain information on abortion morbidity, its data collection may be seriously flawed as to its methodology and findings.[46]

Finally, the report concluded that the studies with the most flaws are those most likely to report positive outcomes.[47] Also, it is likely that even the data currently available "under-represent the extent of the negative psychological aftermath of post abortion."[48]

Appendix One of the report cited and described the findings of ninety studies from 1963–87, which indicated that post abortion psychological problems occur in a significant number of women.[49] Reading through this appendix was sobering, to say the least, as the different doctors and researchers stressed the serious psychological problems they found resulting from abortion. Here are a few examples of what they said:

Joy (1985):
Clinical report indicating a significant number of women are requesting counseling for a depression problem found to be an expression of unresolved grief over a prior abortion. Most women who chose abortion did so in haste and relative social isolation.

Lodl, McGettigan, and Bucy (1985):
There is a reluctance to call attention to negative consequences of abortion for fear of being seen as providing support to anti-abortion and pro-natalist pressure groups.

Reardon (1986):
Of 230 women studied, the majority felt "forced" to have an abortion; 83 percent felt "rushed" to make decision; 71 percent believed their abortion counselors were biased; 80 percent suffered chronic negative psychological sequelae; 19 percent reported suicidal ideation; and 20 percent reported chemical dependencies.

Speckhard (1986):
Found abortion a stresser event for most women interviewed and that delayed psychological complications occurred for most of the women studied five to ten years post abortion. Eighty-five percent were surprised by the intensity of their negative emotional reactions. Eighty-one percent felt victimized by their abortions.

Wall (1986):
Examined 34 women post abortion. Majority reported chronic emotional problems in the abortion aftermath, including guilt, depression, alcohol and drug abuse, difficulty in relationships, and anxiety in subsequent pregnancies. Twenty-six percent reported making some suicidal gestures since their abortion.

Hittner (1987):
Women with children are more likely to be negatively affected by abortion. Delayed grief was also found. . . . These findings raise questions about the beliefs that only a few women experience post abortion emotional difficulties.

In conclusion, the promoters of abortion may claim that abortion is safe, but it is simply not true.

Fraud and Consequence: The Kinsey Research and Planned Parenthood

How Deception Changed a Nation

One of the premises of modern sex education is that lack of sound information is a major cause of our problems. If kids are given the right information, they will act accordingly in light of what's right for them. But not only is this assumption wrong, kids today aren't even getting sound information. They are getting *distortions* seemingly designed to undermine traditional morality in support of sexual freedom. What's worse, sex education courses are often based on the evolutionary premise that man is only a higher form of animal and that "traditional morality" is something unhealthy and repressive. This view of man and morality regulates the nature of sex education so that education about sex actually becomes the vehicle through which sexual immorality is encouraged. In this chapter we will show why much of what teens and preteens are taught is part of an agenda designed to lead them into sexual activity.

THE KINSEY RESEARCH

It is difficult to overestimate the impact of the original Kinsey Research upon modern sex education. Much of the influence of Planned Parenthood can be traced to the "scientific" findings of Alfred Kinsey and his group in the 1940s and 50s. In fact, this work continues today through the Kinsey Institute for Research in Sex, Gender, and Reproduction at the Indiana University campus: "This institute is currently expanding its national role more than ever— entering biomedical research, initiating and participating in conferences, distributing syndicated sex advice columns and providing massive sex information resources on an international scale."[1]

"No man in modern times has shaped public attitudes to, and perceptions of, human sexuality more than the late Alfred C. Kinsey."[2] Kinsey's major texts were *Sexual Behavior in the Human Male* (1948) and *Sexual Behavior in the Human Female* (1953), both with Wardell B. Pomeroy and Clyde E. Martin. "More than any other documents in history, they have shaped Western society's beliefs and understanding about what human sexuality is. They have defined what people *allegedly* do sexually, thereby, establishing what is allegedly *normal*. Their impact on attitudes, subsequent developments in sexual behavior, politics, law, sex education and even religion has been immense though this is not generally realized by the public today."[3] (For example, the pervasive influence of the *Playboy* empire may be directly attributable to the transformation in perspective that Kinsey's research wrought on an impressionable young Hugh Hefner).[4]

But Hugh Hefner was certainly not the only person influenced by reading the Kinsey Research. We have received numerous letters from individuals who have commented that it was the initial Kinsey research that helped them see that all sexual behavior is relative. They told us how it encouraged them to abandon their moral upbringing and engage in sexual promiscuity. Steve wrote:

> My first exposure to Kinsey was absolutely liberating. Finally, here was scientific proof that I could do whatever I wanted. Nothing was really wrong, and there were no reasons not to have all the sex I wanted. I even tried homosexual relations—and happily concluded I was bisexual.
>
> Although I am now married with two children, I continue to have an exciting life with several male lovers. My wife is unaware of this; nevertheless, I find it tremendously invigorating to our relationship.

What Kinsey taught was that all sexual behaviors, including those considered deviant, were merely gradations on a "normal" scale. Because man is an animal and moral values are relative, all types of sexual behavior can be considered normal. But if the entire spectrum of sexuality is normal, then "restrictive" sexuality can be seen as the product of repressive social codes. Monogamous heterosexuality is, more or less, only a product of cultural inhibitions and social conditioning.[5]

Unfortunately, thirty-five years after Kinsey's research, his "conclusions have become, to some extent, a self-fulfilling prophecy. They are the basis for much that is taught in sex education and for an ongoing agenda to engineer public attitudes about human sexuality."[6]

> A sex education "establishment" in the United States is well on the way to introducing full-blown Kinseyan philosophy into the nation's schools, via control of sex education programming. (The distillate of Kinsey philosophy . . . is that every type of sexual activity is natural and thus normal, and should begin as early in life as possible.) How has this control been achieved? Quite simply, by gaining the power to set the accreditation guidelines for the only formal university based degree programs for human sexuality educators. In other words, many, if not most, of today's professional sex educators are schooled and graduated in Kinsey's philosophy.[7]

Until recently, hardly anyone suspected that Kinsey's conclusions might have been wrong—let alone biased, fraudulent, or implicated in criminal activity. The standard text *Masters and Johnson on Sex and Human Loving* (1988) cites Kinsey as if his conclusions were valid: "The Kinsey Reports were based on extensive face-to-face interviews with 12,000 people from all segments of the population, and the findings were often startling. For instance, 37 percent of American men were reported to have had at least one homosexual experience to the point of orgasm after the age of puberty; 40 percent of husbands had been unfaithful to their wives."[8]

But this trust in Kinsey has proven false. In *Kinsey, Sex and Fraud*, Dr. Judith Reisman and others document the extent of bias and fraud that Kinsey and his co-workers have foisted upon the public. In the foreword Dr. John H. Court writes about Kinsey's methods:

> Starting from uncertain data, reported with surprising levels of inaccuracy, generalizing well beyond the limits allowed by the inherent bias in the samples, Kinsey is shown to have spawned a whole movement dedicated to conveying a radical view of sexuality which is fast becoming the norm. To the advocates of homosexual liberation and pedophilia, this presents no problems, but rather a springboard for advocacy. . . . Perhaps we should not be surprised when we see the headway that has been made by gay activists and by pedophiles in shaping public opinion. Yet it is surprising that so many apparently responsible professionals can accept the Kinsey findings so uncritically even at a time when the STD's, and especially AIDS, are making the risks of promiscuity and anal sex so enormous. We cannot afford to rest our understanding of human sexual response on false data. The implications are just too great.[9]

Reisman and her associates revealed the following about the god-father of the modern sexual revolution:

- Criminal sexual experimentation upon children "formed the basis of Kinsey's conclusions on childhood sexual potential. The results of these experiments are the basis for beliefs on childhood sexuality held and taught by academic sexologists today."[10]
- Animal sexual behavior was an appropriate model for human sexual behavior. "Nowhere are Kinsey's interpretations more obvious than in his comparisons of human and animal behavior. Behaviors historically condemned by society are described as normal and justified by 'normal mammalian practices.'"[11] Even sexual relations between humans and animals were granted a measure of dignity.[12]
- Normal heterosexual relations were relegated to an inferior position along the sexual spectrum.[13] Bisexuality was the more "balanced" sexual orientation for "normal uninhibited" persons.[14]
- Kinsey's allegedly "scientific" research was based on highly unrepresentative population samples: "Kinsey revealed little about the exact composition of his total male interviewee sample, which should have been representative of the population of the United States. It is now clear that it contained inappropriate numbers of sex offenders, paedophiles and exhibitionists, and a significant portion of it (perhaps 25 percent) consisted of prison inmates. Even those persons who volunteered for Kinsey's research were shown to have been biased toward the sexually unconventional. Kinsey knew this, but concealed the evidence."[15]

Apparently, Kinsey hoped his own agenda—amoral sexuality—would undermine traditional Christian moral values through a consistent "hammering at Judeo-Christian legal and moral codes."[16] For example, besides citing his "findings" of high rates of homosexuality and adultery among males, his Female Report indicated that premarital sexual intercourse was helpful to women in their emotional, social, and sexual adjustment. Avoidance of premarital intercourse was a potential source of damaging inhibitions that could bring problems to marriage.[17] Further, even children were held to be sexual beings from infancy, and "they could, and should, have pleasurable and beneficial sexual interaction with adult 'partners' who could lead them into the proper techniques of fulfilling sexual activity."[18]

But in drawing all these conclusions, Kinsey and his co-workers were apparently only manipulating data to justify their own biases:

> There is good evidence that Kinsey's research was designed to provide a scientific base for his pre-existing radical, sexual ideology: his coworkers were chosen *for their bias;* biased samples were *knowingly* used; unwarranted conclusions were drawn from data presented; methods are sometimes obscured, sometimes flawed; some data are contradictory; there is a prior history of deception in other scientific endeavors; Kinsey has dissembled [concealed intentions] in medical literature; Kinsey co-authors have knowingly misrepresented their data in subsequent publications; criminal experimentation has been the prime source of Kinsey's childhood sexuality data."[19]

In conclusion, "In the case of Kinsey's sex research, there is strong (we believe compelling) evidence of fraud, which would make this research the most egregious example of scientific deception in this century."[20]

Unfortunately, we live in a nation today where children are frequently the victims of social policies, family breakdowns, and sexual exploitation. The extent of Kinsey's responsibility for the current conditions is unknown, but certainly his advocacy of adult/child sexual relations and the normalcy of homosexuality bears a significant responsibility for undergirding current liberal social attitudes that have betrayed children. Kinsey's "data" is not only an encouragement to pedophiles even today, his own experiments with children were, according to Dr. Reisman and her colleagues, *criminal.*

> With respect to Kinsey's experimental child sex research, it will become obvious that this involved the actual perpetration of illegal and sometimes violent sex acts on children. . . . If Kinsey's science is flawed, then today's children are among his prime victims, which is ironic in a way because children also were the prime victims in the live sex experiments which took place in the 1940s and which form the basis of many Kinsey conclusions.
>
> It is Kinsey's work which established the notion of "normal" childhood sexual desire. This "scientific" fact about children provides justification for pedophiles and a "scientific" basis for the children-can-enjoy-sex-with-peers (then with adults) movement that clearly exists within the sexology and sex education establishments today. Children are victims here also because they are not in a position to take part in the debate over the scientific evidence for their own sexuality. They are not in a position to analyze Kinsey's research data that are used to argue the case that they can benefit from, and have a *right* to sex with adults. The debate also is being directed to some extent by those who, while seeming to champion "children's rights," are on record as desiring legal sanction for adult sex with children. . . . One requirement necessary for legitimization of adult/child sexual activity has been met with Kinsey's "demonstration" that children can and should have active sex lives. Steps toward meeting the other requirement have just recently (1988) begun to be discussed openly, with the proposition from a "nationally

recognized expert on sex offenders" that "pedophilia . . . may be a sexual orientation rather than a sexual deviation."[21]

Thus, the growing pedophile movement in our country, as represented by the homosexual national man/boy love association (NAMBLA) and other groups, often cite Kinsey's work as justification for its existence and activities. "Another group grateful to Kinsey is the proliferating paedophile movement, which justifies its advocacy of adult sexual relations with children by quoting Kinsey's child sexuality findings. Tom O'Carroll, an active paedophile, chairperson of the International Organization PIE (Paedophile Information Exchange) and author of *Pedophilia: the Radical Case* . . . cites Kinsey's research (correctly) as [allegedly] supporting the harmlessness of adult/child sexual interaction."[22]

As a result of Kinsey's research, homosexuality is also increasingly taught as a normal lifestyle option in sex education courses today. Children throughout America learn that

> Kinsey established that 10 percent of American males are "normally" homosexual. In the Los Angeles school district, for example, a program was introduced in 1984 called "Project 10" (after Kinsey)—a gay and lesbian counseling service for youth. Described in the publication *United Teacher* as "a model for school districts throughout the United States," this program offers books featuring stories on homosexual love-making (claimed to be written by children) and is an attempt to help children "accept" their homosexuality, as well as their sexual potential.[23]

The fact that Kinsey's statistics on the prevalence of homosexuality in society were grossly in error has somehow been ignored by modern sex educators. They continually cite the 10 percent figure. But Kinsey claimed only that 10 percent of white American males are "more or less exclusively homosexual" for at least three years between the ages of sixteen and fifty-five—and even this was probably false when written. The true figure for lifelong homosexuality today is probably 1 to 4 percent at best.[24]

Even incest can find justification in the Kinsey research. Pomeroy argues, "It is time to admit that incest need not be a perversion or a symptom of mental illness. . . . Incest between . . . children and adults . . . can sometimes be beneficial."[25] Leading sex researcher John Money of Johns Hopkins argues, "A childhood sexual experience, such as being the partner of a relative or of an older person, need not necessarily affect the child adversely."[26]

Further, the Kinsey research has fueled the multibillion dollar pornography industry in the United States—with all its enormous consequences—and in addition, "the Kinsey studies, as much as pornography, shaped the context in which the Supreme Court responded to the obscenity issue."[27] Further, "if the legitimate pornography industry is, in a sense, another Kinsey legacy, then its leaders are clearly grateful. According to Christie Hefner, in the 1960s the Playboy Foundation became the major research sponsor of the Masters and Johnson Institute and made the initial grant to establish an Office of Research Services of the Sex Information and Education Counsel of the U.S. (SIECUS). The latter organization is heavily involved in the incorporation of Kinsey's basic sexual philosophy into school sex education programs."[28]

The average American has little understanding of the horrendous consequences of the multibillion dollar pornography industry in society—ranging from child abuse and the degradation of women to the spreading of AIDS and other STDs. Christian organizations around the country have received thousands of letters from individuals who "innocently" became trapped into a pornographic lifestyle by exposure to "soft porn" magazines such as *Playboy*. Many of these individuals later became addicted to frightening forms of sexual expression. This placed their own health and life at risk—or that of others, even young children.

Yet the more enlightened in our nation would have us believe that pornography carries virtually no social consequences and must be defended at all costs as a form of "freedom of speech." Tell that to Nick. He recalls:

> I never intended to become addicted, but I found myself being compelled by something more powerful than my will to resist. At first, it was just looking at magazines. Then, it progressed to X-rated movies, including child porn and sadomasochistic stuff, even snuff films. After that, I began having strong desires for sex with children. I hurt several of them.
>
> It seems that every sexual experience I had soon burned out, and I needed a stronger or more bizarre experience to retain the excitement. Finally, after molesting three dozen children (I even killed two for a sexual thrill), I was caught and sentenced to life in the Federal Penitentiary. I have been raped four times in my first two years.
>
> Don't tell me pornography has no consequences. I'll put a gun to your head.

Yet incredibly today, for many sex therapists and educators, pornographic magazines and movies are actually supplied to people seeking counseling assistance as "tools" to help their sexual "dysfunctions."

When we visited the SIECUS headquarters in New York, talked with staff, and examined the materials for sale, as well as their extensive sex library, it became obvious that SIECUS, too, was a powerful governmental arm for promoting liberal/Kinseyan sexual attitudes in society.[29]

What's worse, most scientists involved in the creation of the Kinsey findings are today living and functioning as influential researchers, scholars, lecturers, writers, experts on sexuality, courtroom witnesses, and authorities in sex education. They continue to espouse the Kinsey data as factual science when it appears to be little more than fraudulent social engineering. Why these individuals have not renounced Kinsey and apologized to the nation is a question that can be answered only by them. As Dr. Reisman observes, "Fraud is a serious charge. It calls for re-evaluation of the greatest single human sexuality research project ever undertaken and an assessment of the damage it may have caused to society. And since Kinsey co-authors Pomeroy and Gibhard are still well-known and influential sexologists, and the Kinsey Institute presumably still houses all Kinsey's original data, it calls for a response from these sources."[30]

PLANNED PARENTHOOD

Planned Parenthood is, in some respects, another legacy of the Kinsey research. Until recently, it was a largely ignored or maligned institution that barely scraped by. But in the last two decades it has become one of the most powerful social organizations for disseminating almost everything that is wrong in modern attitudes toward sexuality and sex education.

When we visited the national headquarters of Planned Parenthood in New York to gather research materials, we were startled at the almost Machiavellian atmosphere. It was a bit like a minimum security prison. Locks, restrictions, and security guards were strategically placed—there was even a lock on the library, and no entrance was granted without special permission.

The influence of Planned Parenthood programs in modern sex

education is dramatic. "In spite of this prevalence of sex education, Planned Parenthood has targeted various states so that schools would be mandated to teach comprehensive sex education. In its most recent 'Five-Year Plan,' Planned Parenthood Federation of America commits to increase to fifteen the number of states with mandatory K–12 sexuality educational curricula. . . . As states are considering how to resolve the problem of teenage pregnancy, they tend to be strongly influenced by the Planned Parenthood concept of what sex education should be."[31]

Further, "family planning proponents often insist that their programs do not promote promiscuity, and therefore they are not at all responsible for the teen sexuality crisis. Yet, Planned Parenthood listed 'universal reproductive freedom' as its major goal in its Five-Year Plan for 1976–80. As early as 1963, then-president of Planned Parenthood, Alan Guttmacher (after whom the organization's research arm was named) acknowledged that contraceptive information for teens would bring about an increase in sexual promiscuity."[32] Indeed, the work of Planned Parenthood has helped to bring about:

- General social acceptance of teenage birth control and sex outside of marriage
- An epidemic of sexually transmitted diseases
- Millions of teenage pregnancies and abortion on demand—regardless of parents' wishes
- The increasing denigration of parenthood and the family
- Homosexuality as a legitimate sexual lifestyle option
- Increasing social engineering and perhaps even increasing openness to eugenics

Planned Parenthood, like the Kinsey research, has become a major force for social evil.

> Supreme Court decisions in federal policy have basically made the United States a vast laboratory for Planned Parenthood's ideas these past twenty years. Abortion has been available on demand until term. . . . 1.5 million teenagers per year, and maybe more since 1983, have been enrolled in birth control programs; 150 school-based clinics have opened; media of all kinds have glorified pro-birth control sexual ethics. Major victories for traditional family values have been few and far between. . . . Planned Parenthood's grand experiment has truly proven, as George Grant has written, a grand illusion. What a tragedy it is that our nation has been forced to pay the price of so many broken lives, so many wounded families."[33]

For example, those who read George Grant's *Grand Illusion: The*

Legacy of Planned Parenthood or Robert Marshall and Charles Donovan's *Blessed Are the Barren: The Social Policy of Planned Parenthood* or Douglas R. Scott's *Inside Planned Parenhood* will be shocked at what they discover. Planned Parenthood is truly a "sensually fueled death machine that has taken on world wide proportions."[34] Dr. Bernard Nathanson, a former leader in the abortion industry, who personally presided over sixty thousand abortions, comments about *Blessed Are the Barren*: "This encyclopedic, monumental work is a veritable resource handbook for anyone interested in the sinister workings of the infinitely evil Planned Parenthood empire. It should be required reading for those who understand the malevolent dynasty of the House of Sanger. I recommend this book without reservation or qualification."[35]

John Cardinal O'Connor writes, "This is a sickening book, terribly difficult for any reader who wants to believe in the integrity of the political system, the judiciary, the legal and medical professions, the decency and reasonableness of the people in a whole variety of influential positions. The story of deceit the book relates is devastating."[36]

But perhaps the legacy of Planned Parenthood is not all that surprising, considering its founders. For example, the founding mother of birth control, Margaret Sanger, was the originator of Planned Parenthood.[37] Sanger hated Christianity. She supported political assassination and leftist movements in general, where she "learned the propaganda techniques that were later to stand her in such good stead."[38] She accepted "open marriage" and engaged in sex freely, whether single or married. She even claimed that "the marriage bed is the most degenerating influence of the social order. . . a decadent institution, a reactionary development of the sex instinct."[39] Sanger was also heavily involved in the occult. "Biographer Madeline Gray has written that Sanger sought 'poise and surcease for her recurrent depression through astrology, numerology, sex, religious cults. . . .'; [she] attended seances; and [she] was a member of the Rosicrucian Society. . . . Sanger believed she had undergone numerous reincarnations."[40]

Regardless, the impact of Planned Parenthood has been unmistakable:

> If the world needs more food, Planned Parenthood proposes to kill more children or sterilize couples. To cope with sexual desires, eliminate the consequences (children), because curbing sexual desire is impossible. More venereal diseases, rely upon antibiotics because chastity does not work. Fidelity is bothersome. Take the Pill, get sterilized. If killing a child is morally bothersome, simply redefine the baby out of existence. If the family is breaking down in the wake of the contraceptive-clad sexual revolt, appropriate more money for government day care. Faced with growing poverty, abort (kill), contracept, or sterilize the poor. Johnny and Jane cannot read, never mind, give them condoms and the Pill before they propagate any more of their like.

> French philosopher Etienne Gilson once said that "Philosophy always buries its undertakers." Applying this adage to the present situation, we might say that the Planned Parenthood movement in all its social manifestations is its own best funeral director. It believes in death, it inflicts death; let this movement have what it has given others.[41]

13

The Dangers of Homosexuality:
Medical and Social Concerns

The Tragic Consequences of the Homosexual Lifestyle

> *Many gays reject morality, offering any one of a variety of reasons, rational and emotional, for doing so. But there's a simpler, darker reason why many gays choose to live without morality: as ideologies go, amorality is . . . convenient. And the mortal enemy of that convenience is the value judgment.*
>
> *It quickly became clear to us that urban gays assumed a general consensus to the effect that everyone has the right to behave just as he pleases. . . . Everyone was to decide what was "right for him"—in effect, to make up the rules as he went along. In fact, they boiled it down to a single axiom: I can do whatever I want, and you can go to perdition. . . .*
>
> *We found that in the gay press this doctrine had hardened into stone.*
>
> Homosexual authors Kirk and Madsen,
> *After the Ball*

In late 1992 we received a call from an irate trucker who "wanted somebody to know what was going on along the roads of America" and why something had to be done about it. He felt like Lot in the Old Testament.

In the last five years this Christian man had been propositioned no less than three hundred times by homosexuals at rest areas and even at truck stops: ten times more often than by women. At rest stops, homosexuals would rub themselves as he walked by, grab his genitals, or sit in provocative postures on the hood of his truck. He was sick of it and wanted to know what he could do—short of using a police stick—to defend himself.

We had to tell him there was nothing legal he could do, that this was a symptom of our culture's acceptance of homosexuality and its increasing militancy. At least he could share the gospel with men who desperately needed to hear it—because given AIDS, men so bold might not be living much longer anyway.

The information in this chapter should not be construed as an attack upon homosexuals individually. The response of the church to homosexual persons must be a compassionate one because they have been created in God's image and because Christ died for them. As such, they have innate dignity and worth. However, the church must also have the courage to share the truth with homosexuals. The Bible does teach that homosexuality is a sin and that homosexuals, like unrepentant sexual sinners among the heterosexual population, will not enter the kingdom of heaven.

We recognize that not every homosexual person has the same lifestyle in terms of the potential for sexual excess. But when examined as a whole, the homosexual lifestyle is anything but healthy. It is our hope that this chapter will lead those who read it, whether gay or straight, to recognize the dangers in that lifestyle and to take appropriate personal action.

In 1986 both the American Public Health Association and the American Psychological Association testified before the U.S. Supreme Court that "no significant data show that engaging in . . . oral and anal sex, results in mental or physical dysfunction."[1] The claim of many homosexuals is that their lifestyle is joyous, creative, fulfilling, and loving. But the facts do not support such a view.

According to some preliminary research of Dr. Paul Cameron, homosexuals as a population may have a significantly shortened lifespan irrespective of AIDS—approximately forty-five years.[2]

> On its face, the consistency of the median age of death for gays indexed by the obituaries of seven independent homosexual journals over an eight year period [three thousand individuals], suggests an average life-span locating in the early to mid-40s if AIDS fails to intervene, late 30s if it does. . . . This seems a tad discordant with van den Haag's assertion that "homosexuality does not shorten life" or Bancroft's 1988 contention in the *British Medical Journal* that it is "compatible with full health."[3]

Additional research conducted in 1992 expanded the data base to 5,371 obituaries from sixteen American homosexual journals, which were compared to a large sample of obituaries from regular newspapers:

The median age of death for homosexuals, however, was virtually the same nationwide [39 to 42 years]—and, overall, less than 2 percent survived to old age. If AIDS was the cause of death, the median age was 39. For the 588 gays who died of something other than AIDS, the median age of death was 42 and 9 percent died old. The 106 lesbians had a median age of death of 45 and 26 percent died old. . . . Heart attacks, cancer and liver failure were exceptionally common.[4]

In the material to follow we will briefly examine the relationship of homosexuality to (1) suicide, (2) pornography, (3) sexually transmitted diseases other than AIDS, (4) child molestation, (5) social conscience, (6) criminality, and (7) self-deception. Insofar as the "sexual revolution" has undergirded homosexuality, all these can be seen as further consequences of liberal attitudes toward sexuality in general.

HOMOSEXUALITY AND SUICIDE

Even before AIDS the incidence of suicide among homosexuals was above the norm. "Suicide attempts are significantly higher among homosexuals than among others—for example, 3% for white non-homosexual males, 18% for white homosexual males."[5]

Homosexuals much more frequently contemplate suicide (in [one study] 27% of male heterosexuals vs. 46% of gays and 34% of female normals vs. 56% of lesbians reported contemplating suicide at least once). As would be expected, homosexuals much more frequently attempt suicide (in [the same study] 5% of normal males versus 19% of gays and 10% of heterosexual females versus 21% of lesbians reported at least one suicide attempt)."[6]

Homosexual John Rechy observes concerning the world of promiscuous homosexuality, "Once chosen, it's a world that carries him to the pinnacle of sexual freedom—the high that only outlaw sex can bring—as well as to the abyss of suicide."[7]

But in light of the AIDS epidemic, matters have degenerated greatly. For example, "according to a New York City study, AIDS patients were committing suicide at a far higher rate than the general population, and at a higher rate than among people with other fatal diseases. . . . These data indicated that men with AIDS were *36 times* more likely to commit suicide than the entire population of men 20 to 59 years old, and *66 times* more likely than the general population."[8] In addition, the *Journal of the American Medical Association* ran an article in 1988 that further explored the problem.[9]

Unfortunately, "it was not uncommon for someone to kill himself following the discovery of a positive result."[10] Dr. Patrick Dixon goes so far as to state, "Suicide is a common terminal event with people with AIDS—usually early in the illness—but also tragically in people who have had a positive test result, especially if counseling afterwards was poor."[11] But in addition, "a small but growing number are also committing suicide because they [only] *fear* they have AIDS."[12]

Further, suicide among teenage homosexuals is so common that the "Report of the Secretary's Task Force on Youth Suicide" has suggested an ironic solution—that society more fully accept and encourage homosexuality as a preventative to teenage suicides.[13]

HOMOSEXUALITY AND PORNOGRAPHY

Pornography apparently plays a significant or major role in the life of the average homosexual. Roger Montgomery, a former homosexual prostitute who became a Christian prior to his death from AIDS, observed, "Although it is not widely spoken of or acknowledged, pornography plays a prominent place in the life of every homosexual. Indeed, homosexuals bear a great burden of responsibility for the promotion of pornography in America, including child pornography."[14] Citing a survey of 4,340 adults in five American cities in 1983 and 842 adults in Dallas in 1984, Paul Cameron concludes that homosexuals "are prodigious consumers of pornography."[15]

HOMOSEXUALITY AND SEXUALLY TRANSMITTED DISEASES OTHER THAN AIDS

"According to Drs. Edward J. Artnak and James J. Cerda, writing in the medical journal *Current Concepts in Gastroenterology,* the male homosexual 'is responsible for the majority of new cases of sexually transmitted diseases.' The Centers for Disease Control have reported that approximately 50 percent of new cases of syphilis occur in the homosexual population."[16]

According to other research homosexuals are:

- Fourteen times more apt ever to have had syphilis
- Three times more apt ever to have had gonorrhea
- Three times more apt ever to have had genital warts
- Eight times more apt ever to have had hepatitis
- Three times more apt ever to have had lice
- Five times more apt ever to have had scabies

- Thirty times more apt ever to have had an infection from penile contact
- Hundreds of times more apt to have had oral infection from penile contact
- Over five thousand times more apt to have had AIDS.[17]

Below we will present additional evidence of the incidence of STDs in the homosexual population and reveal how such diseases are spreading into the heterosexual population. In essence, increasing social acceptance of homosexuality is resulting in increasing STD infection of nonhomosexuals.

According to various studies, approximately 70 to 80 percent of homosexuals have reported having a sexually transmitted disease.[18] In the August 1985 issue of *The Nebraska Medical Journal* four researchers wrote an article on "Sexual Orientation and Sexually Transmitted Disease." They concluded: "Bi-/homosexuals of both genders (4.4 percent of the same) reported higher lifetime rates for most of the STDs and admitted to higher rates of deliberate infection of others than their heterosexual counterparts."[19] Further,

> Homosexuals account for about triple of their proportionate share of STDs. . . . Since people do not always know the sexual histories or current sexual habits of their partners, the possibility that homosexual activity accounts for an even greater proportion of STDs than reported in Table One is considerable. Since a large fraction of homosexual practitioners go "both ways," homosexuals constitute an important vector of infection for the entire society. Diseases ranging from typhoid fever to the various forms of hepatitis may be transmitted sexually. . . . The extent to which persons who engage in homosexual acts decrease collective health would seem to warrant substantial attention. Denver's STD clinic recently reported that about 41 percent of their gonorrhea case load was contributed by homosexual men."[20]

An article in the *New England Journal of Medicine* su;mmarized the findings of ten researchers, among them four M.D.s and four Ph.D.s: "We found that in men, a history of receptive anal intercourse (related to homosexual behavior) was strongly associated with the occurrence of anal cancer (relative risk, 33.1; 95 percent confidence interval, 4.0 to 272.1). . . . We conclude that homosexual behavior in men is a risk factor for anal cancer."[21]

The Annals of Internal Medicine, contained an article that concluded,

> In addition to gonorrhea and syphilis, both of which may develop primarily at anorectal or pharyngeal sites, a number of conditions, including *Neisseria meningitides* urethritis, non specific urethritis, anorectal herpes, condyloma acuminatum, amebiasis, giardiasis, shigellosis, typhoid fever, enterobiasis,

and hepatitis A and B, have been identified as being transmitted by male homosexual contact. Protologic complications of anal intercourse include allergic reactions to anal lubricants, prolapsed hemorrhoids, anal fistulas, and fissures. Rectosigmoid tears may result from fist, forearm, and foreign body penetration of the bowel.[22]

This article indicated that a recent report from the CDC revealed that almost half the male patients with syphilis claimed homosexual or bi-sexual contacts.[23] It noted that analrectal and pharyngeal gonorrhea "are particularly prevalent in homosexual men."[24] It also discussed the physical problems encountered with "fisting:" "Several cases of peritonitis resulting from rectosigmoid tears after insertion of a fist or even a forearm for sexual gratification are seen in the emergency rooms of hospitals in San Francisco and other cities each year. . . . Trauma to the external genitalia may occur during homosexual intercourse. Streptococcal pyoderma has been reported as a complication of fellatio. . . . Penile edema . . . may also be seen in patients who habitually utilize penile rings."[25] The author of this article was concerned that correct diagnosis of STDs be made "to prevent the development of serious complications, for example, amebic hepatic or brain abscesses."[26] Further, other homosexually transmitted diseases include typhoid fever, enterobiasis, and campylobacter infections.[27]

But what was perhaps most surprising about this article was the attitude that "physicians can best help their homosexual patients by accepting them and their relationships non-judgmentally and by understanding their special health needs," and, if this were not possible, "referral to another physician is indicated."[28] One wonders what the word *help* means today when even a physician (one who is supposed to help heal) offers "non-judgmental" counsel concerning a lifestyle that is so destructive. Is the attitude of some physicians today toward "helping" homosexuals that of merely treating their diseases while saying nothing at all about the very behavior causing the diseases?

HOMOSEXUALITY AND CHILD MOLESTATION

Homosexuals often argue that child molestation occurs much more frequently among heterosexuals than homosexuals—as if this somehow justified sodomy with young boys. Whereas this is true statistically, it is not true proportionately, because homosexuals have a much higher rate of molestation:

> The most recent review of the child molestation literature as it appears in medical and psychological journals concluded that between 25 and 40 percent of all recorded child molestation was homosexual. . . . In the Family Research Institute's national random survey of 4,340 adults, we found that about a third of those who reported having been molested were homosexually molested. . . . The *Los Angeles Times* poll of 2,628 adults (8/26/85) reported that about a third of those molested as children had been homosexually molested.[29]

In one survey titled "World's Recent Literature Regarding Child Molestation," the ratio of heterosexual/homosexual assault on children was given as follows: "About 42 percent of all victims of molestation were assaulted by those who practice homosexuality. Homosexual practitioners are at least 12 times and probably 18 times (with the bi-sexual correction) more apt to incorporate minors into their sexual practices than heterosexuals are."[30]

In other words, homosexuals who comprise approximately 1–4 percent of the world's population are responsible for between 30 and 50 percent of all recorded molestations. In addition, homosexual teachers "have committed between a quarter to four-fifths of all molestation of pupils!"[31] Apparently, this high incidence of child molestation among the homosexual population is accounted for on the basis of the overprizing of youth in conjunction with the overpowering sexual lust many homosexuals experience.

Other studies may also reveal that many homosexuals have sexual relations with the young. The original Kinsey study claimed that 37 percent of gays and 2 percent of lesbians admitted to sexual relations with under seventeen-year olds; the second Kinsey study said one-fourth of gays admitted to homosexual relationships with under sixteen-year olds. In that much of Kinsey's research was based on unrepresentative samples, these figures may be suspect. Nevertheless, in the *Gay Report*, 23 percent of gays and 6 percent of lesbians admitted to sexual interaction with youth less than sixteen years of age.[32]

Recent discussions with a number of psychiatrists who counsel homosexuals, as well as conversations with former homosexuals, indicate the possibility that at least 75 percent and as much as 90 percent of all homosexuals had been actively recruited into the homosexual lifestyle through sexual molestation by an older man.

> While no one study is definitive, taken together the literature constitutes the bulk of what social science has to add to common sense in formulating social policy regarding homosexuals' interaction with children. . . . [In addition] homosexuals' activists are the driving force behind the North American Man-Boy Love Association and the Childhood Sensuality Circle. . . . Empirical research to date corroborates the common opinion that homosexuals have a considerably greater propensity to recruit, solicit, and molest children.[33]

But some tell us we must not discriminate against those who prefer to have sex with children, whether homosexual or heterosexual. Perhaps we should all follow the socially enlightened example of the University of Massachusetts at Amhurst, which has apparently revised its nondiscrimination code. The earlier Affirmative Action and Non-Discrimination Policy had excluded "persons whose sexual orientation includes minor children as the sex object." According to the Family Research Report, it no longer does.[34]

HOMOSEXUALITY AND SOCIAL CONSCIENCE

The extreme lack of social conscience found in some homosexuals might also be labeled the Gaetan Dugas syndrome—after Gaetan Dugas who, upon learning he had AIDS, set out to infect as many men as possible. We mentioned "revenge sex" earlier. We conclude that (1) homosexual anger, (2) human nature, and (3) our own research lead us to believe the incidence is greater than many people suspect. It is not surprising that many of those who are desperate, who are amoral, and who hate themselves or a society which is "permitting" them to die by the hundreds of thousands might be expected to take personal revenge. "Often the homosexual's attitude has been 'I'm going to die anyway. I might as well take somebody with me.'"[35] One AIDS-infected person claimed that he had infected seventy patients with his own blood.[36] In addition, many threats or violent tactics have been reported against those homosexuals consider their enemies.[37]

According to the *Dallas Gay News* (May 20, 1983) homosexual Robert Schwab, former president of the Texas Human Rights Foundation and a homosexual activist dying of AIDS, stated the following:

"There has come the idea that if research money is not forthcoming at a certain level by a certain date, that all gay males should give blood. . . . If it takes threatening and perhaps giving blood to get us the money. . . . Whatever action is required to get national attention is valid. If that includes blood terrorism, so be it."[38]

Even some hospitals have apparently been threatened by homosexuals with donating AIDS-contaminated blood if they did not give in to homosexual concerns.[39] If homosexuals as a population have higher incidences of deliberately infecting their partners, knowing they have various sexually transmitted diseases, and even AIDS, it would seem that anything is possible. One would think that the person who knows he is dying from a terribly painful, lethal disease, who is himself the victim of a self-centered neurosis and who is angry and bitter against society might become a passive killer without a great deal of provocation.[40]

The attitude of Troy Perry, founder of the homosexual Metropolitan Community Churches, is typical: "I presume we've all been exposed to the virus. I just take the attitude that every gay man has been exposed to the virus, but I refuse to go down there [to take a test] and have my name in some computer somewhere."[41] Elsewhere *California* magazine (July 1983) reported that the homosexual community chose to permit hundreds and probably thousands of its own members to die rather than risk a social backlash against them. If it treats its own people this way, how do we think it will treat those it considers outsiders—or even its enemies?

In North Carolina the law requires HIV positive persons to notify their sex or drug partners. Yet among seventy-four HIV positive patients, only eighteen of 310 sexual partners of the last year were notified. Further, in Los Angeles more than 50 percent of infected men confessed they did not tell one or more of their lovers about their HIV infection. Finally, 7 percent of the Family Research Institutes' random national urban sample of male homo—and bisexuals admitted they had sex merely in order to infect others.[42]

HOMOSEXUALITY AND CRIMINALITY

Until recently, homosexual acts were considered criminal, although the law was rarely enforced. Indeed, in 1988 alone, eighteen more states removed their sodomy laws.[43] This leaves only a handful that retain such laws. But if tens of millions die from AIDS, this will probably force a return to the viewpoint of homosexual acts, and sexual immorality in general, as criminal. What is surprising is that homosexual acts were ever decriminalized in the first place. It is hard to fathom why any lifestyle that has a higher incidence of suicide, promotes pornography, spreads serious sexually transmitted diseases throughout its own population and the rest of society, involves a much higher rate of child molestation, would *not* be considered criminal. Of course, thanks to much of modern psychology, the Kinseys, and Hugh Hefners we live in an age of sexual "enlightenment" and know better.

On January 31, 1986, the American Psychological Association filed an *amicus curiae* brief before the Supreme Court favoring the constitutional protection for consenting homosexual acts among adults, despite an apparent misrepresentation of scientific material to the Supreme Court on behalf of this brief.[44]

When powerful lobbyists and the government itself throw their collective weight behind the public promotion of a sinful lifestyle with serious consequences for individuals both here and in eternity, the church must act to stem the tide. The fact that sodomy laws are now removed from the majority of individual states and that this has happened in the last twenty years gives one an indication of the trend.[45]*

But, further, it appears that homosexuality and its lifestyle actually increases criminal behavior. The Institute for the Scientific Investigation of Sexuality (ISIS) examined the incidence of criminality and social disruption among the homosexual population: "Homosexuals, like others addicted to very bad habits, are a net burden on society."[46] Further, "four major studies allow a comparison of homosexuals with heterosexuals—and all generated results suggesting greater social

---

* The best discussion we have read concerning the importance of recriminalization of homosexuality and what the church and state's position should be is Greg Bahnsen, *Homosexuality: A Biblical View*, chap. 5.

disruption on the part of gays. Saghir and Robbins compared 146 gay volunteers with 78 heterosexuals and reported less stability . . . and more criminality among homosexuals. Bell and Weinberg contrasted 979 volunteer gays with 477 randomly-obtained 'mainly heterosexuals' and found more instability (psychiatric, marital) and more criminality among gays."[47] In addition:

- 62 percent more homosexuals reported regularly getting high on drugs or alcohol. (According to former homosexual prostitute, Roger Montgomery, hard drugs are freely available in gay bars, and widely used among homosexuals. Unfortunately, those with drug habits are much more inclined to commit criminal acts.)
- 31 percent more gays reported at least one auto accident in the past five years.
- 40 percent more gays admitted to deliberately killing or attempting to kill others.
- 557 percent more gays reported having been arrested for a sexual crime.
- 41 percent more gays admitted to shoplifting.
- 67 percent more homosexuals admitted cheating on their income tax.
- Homosexuals more frequently violate positions of public trust for sexual advantage.
- Homosexuals were 62 percent more likely to admit to having sex with children under the age of thirteen.[48]

An ISIS publication claims that "most victims of sex murderers died at the hands of 'gays' and that half of all sex murderers are homosexuals." For example, "In an evaluation of 40 mass murders or serial killers it is claimed, that of 'the mass murders involving sexuality over the past 17 years in the U.S., . . . homosexuals are . . . over represented in these 518 deaths.'"[49] Jeffrey Dahmer is only the latest of several notorious cases. (In 1991 homosexual Donald Harvey was indicted on allegedly murdering at least eighty-seven people.) Further, "Various scholars have reviewed the psychological and sociological literature of the world and have concluded that both gays and lesbians are unusually prone to violence. Among police departments, this belief is so pervasive that particularly gory murders are assumed to be homosexual until proven otherwise. . . . It appears that homosexuals account for about two-thirds of all sexual murders."[50]

This is understandable considering statistics like the following: John Wayne Gacy (twenty-three victims), Patrick Kearney (thirty-two victims), Bruce Davis (twenty-eight victims), Corll-Henley-Brooks (twenty-seven victims), Juan Corona (twenty-five victims). In fact, the

New York Times cites investigating detectives as saying that all these murders were "motivated by a sense of shame after having [homo]sexual relations with their victims."[51]

This should not be so surprising. "If people mix sex and violence, it is reasonable to expect that at times the violence will become homicidal. Gay sex is disproportionately violent sex. . . . Disturbed people do disturbing things. . . . Frequently murderers, on the verge of getting caught, commit suicide. Similarly, many of those intent upon suicide decide to 'take a few with [them]. . . . Those who hold their own lives in lower value are more likely to treat your life casually.'"[52]

In "Homosexuals in the Armed Forces," three researchers indicated that, "Consistent with other studies on the issue, 31 percent of the homosexual versus 4 percent of heterosexual men reported less than honorable discharges."[53] These same researchers indicated that homosexuals are more likely to "(1) expose themselves to biological hazards, (2) participate in socially disruptive sex (e.g., deliberate infection of others, cheating in marriage, obscene phone calls) and (3) frequently report engaging in socially disruptive activities. . . . From the standpoints of individual health, public health and social order, participating in homosexual activity could be viewed as dangerous to society and incompatible with full health."[54] In answering the question, "Is homosexuality compatible with social order," they conclude, "Our new material fell at least three to one against homosexuality, and the set of material from the four older studies fell about four to one against homosexuality."[55]

A little known historical fact may be worthy of mention:

> Gay rights began in Germany at the turn of the century. By 1923 there were over 25 national organizations and 33 periodicals catering to homosexuals, and gays were seeking a political party to carry their lifestyle to power. They threw their weight behind the Nazis and were rewarded with leadership of the Storm Troopers (SA). Over time, Nazi youth organizations and camps became notorious for homosexual molestation. Open homosexuality, pornography, drugs and prostitution turned Berlin into the San Francisco of Europe. Confronting a deteriorating social situation, Hitler betrayed his gay comrades and moved forcefully against homosexuals in 1934. In one of the ironic twists of history, gays became some of the first inmates of the death camps they helped to create.[56]

HOMOSEXUALITY AND SELF-DECEPTION

As noted earlier, Roger Montgomery knew several thousand homosexuals in the span of his period as a homosexual and a homosexual prostitute. He observes, "Self-deception is the reality of the homosexual community."[57] As an illustration he cites the rationalizations of homosexuals in defense of their lifestyle against all scientific fact:

> According to the neurophysiological theory, because the brain is irreversibly "sexed" before birth, post-birth experiences cannot reprogram the brain in an alternate sexual direction. This theory is especially dear to homosexuals because it allegedly offers a "scientific, medical support" to the homosexual lifestyle. Thus they claim that post-birth experiences (such as the sexual molestation of a young boy by an older man) do not influence or alter sexual development in any way. . . . The homosexual community wants us to believe they were born gay in hopes that this would absolve them of personal responsibility, including the responsibility for recruiting children through molestation. Thus, a lack of responsibility for who one is, automatically carries with it the lack of responsibility to change their orientation and behavior.[58]

This unsubstantiated and increasingly discredited argument is used by at least one-third of homosexuals to justify their lifestyle.

Another problem is self-labeling. Because the homosexual orientation is perceived as being so "fixed," the individual who finally comes to "accept" his "nature" and to label himself a homosexual automatically sets in motion a series of subsequent events and changes in his own life: all of which are entirely unnecessary.

In other words, instead of resisting the label and the lifestyle, and seeking spiritual or psychological help to deal with what all the evidence reveals is a genuine problem, the problem is accepted as the essence of what one is and redefined as something "good." Can we imagine a drug addict or alcoholic assuming a similar approach to his or her problem, claiming his or her addiction as good and normal? If homosexuality is so normal, why is it that "when they learn they are homosexual, almost all homosexuals are appalled and depressed by this knowledge?"[59]

What's worse, once the self-diagnosis of being a homosexual is made, the doors swing wide open to the homosexual lifestyle. For many, this self-labeling sears all remnants of earlier inhibition and the person dives into the homosexual lifestyle with all its promiscuity. In other words, the self-labeling itself frequently results in a tragic end.

What is truly ironic is that many social scientists, psychotherapists and "sexologists" actively support the process. Once they diagnose someone as a "primary," or "nuclear" and irremediable homosexual, the person is convinced this is his or her "fate"—his or her true nature has emerged and just cannot be changed. Is it so surprising they plunge headlong into the homosexual lifestyle? Why do these so-called experts not make the same kinds of diagnoses for drug addicts or adulterers?

Dr. Gerhard van den Aardweg describes the initial relief at such self-labeling, but also the ultimate cost:

> Young persons who notice homosexual interests in themselves often go through a miserable time. . . . They may feel ashamed; when the topic of homosexuality is touched upon, they want to hide lest others connect it with them. They suffer in silence; maybe they try to deny or play down their feelings, even to themselves. The moment comes, however, often around the age of 18, when the young person has to face his situation. Then he may conclude, "I am a homosexual."
>
> That can give great relief. The acute tension declines, but a price must be paid. The youngsters hardly ever realize that they have fixed a rather definitive label on themselves with this "self-identification" and assigned themselves to a second-class and in fact excluded status. . . . They inwardly realize that their "being different" is an inferior form of sexuality. . . . The toll for this, however, is the depressing fatalism that is implicit in this newly acquired identity: "I am just that way." The young person does not think, "It is true that I have occasional irregular homosexual feelings, but basically I must have been born the same as anyone else." No, he feels he is a different and inferior creature, who carries a doom: he views himself as tragic."[60]

What is doubly sad about this self-labeling is that the individual is never born homosexual and his fate is hardly sealed; he merely has homosexual "feelings." As Aardweg observes, "A careful analysis of the fantasy and dream life over the whole course of the life of a person with strong homosexual tendencies, [reveals that] one always finds traces of a normal, deeply hidden heterosexual disposition."[61]

In other words, the "true homosexual" is really a heterosexual attempting to, for whatever reason, live a disguise—in fact, a lie. "Strictly speaking, then, 'homosexuals' or 'homophiles' do not exist, any more than in the animal realm; you have only *persons with homosexual inclinations*."[62] Eventually, of course, the self-deception matures to such an extent that the falsehood bears fruit—the myth or half-truth becomes the standard; the *feelings* become the person; the *lie* becomes the reality.

The consequences of self-labeling can reinforce the inferiority feelings that may already exist. An "us" versus "them" mentality develops, a feeling of alienation from the normal world, and a virulent bonding to the community of homosexuals takes place. The deception is now both internalized and externalized. Reality is defined by what one thinks one is inwardly and is confirmed externally by reinforcement through a close-knit homosexual community having similar feelings. Homosexual practices and promiscuity become the standard of "healthy, virile sexuality," and a fortress of social reinforcement is provided to protect the inward condition.

The tragedy of this self-labeling, too often reinforced by the psychotherapeutic community, is wholly unnecessary. As even one psychologist confesses, "As a profession, we cannot claim other than a *major role* in the current move toward legitimization of homosexuality."[63]

> Frequently youngsters who express their probably-not-yet-fixated homoerotic feelings or fantasies are informed by the "experts" that they are homosexuals. That may hit hard and dash whatever hopes were there. I suggest as a preferable reaction to young people who disclose their secret feelings something like this: You may indeed feel that interest in your own sex, but it is still a question of immaturity. By nature, you are not that way. Your heterosexual nature has not yet awakened. What we have to discuss is a personality problem.[64]

The problem with telling somebody that he is a homosexual or encouraging him in that direction is that the person, particularly the impressionable youngster, concludes (often with "expert" encouragement) that only when he begins to live his "real nature" will he be happy. Because his sexual tension or confusion can be intense, it is easy to conclude that the solution lies in pursuing homosexual relationships. Allegedly, he is told, this will solve his problems of sexual identity, loneliness, inferiority feelings, and so on.

But sooner or later the individual frequently realizes that he has adopted a disordered and, in fact, neurotic way of life. His addiction, with all the qualities accompanying an addiction, will continue to increase and his ability and will to change will continue to decrease until he is genuinely chained to the homosexual lifestyle.

Consider the following sentiments of two homosexuals who celebrated the national "coming out day" on the Oprah Winfrey Show,

October 11, 1989. One gay audience member simply observed, "I am who I am."[65] And another, who freely admitted that his being homosexual was "a gradual process," finally came to understand: "I realized throughout all this that I had to come to grips and say, 'Okay. This is the way you are. You can't deny it. You've got to face it.'"[66] Again, such self-labeling is self-defeating. If homosexuals believe they *cannot* change, why should they try? But if, as all the scientific evidence suggests, they *can* change their behavior (even after the damage is done)—how many more can change at the earliest stage of self-labeling?[67]

Many are the problems and dangers involved in the homosexual lifestyle. We don't think that as a society we can claim we genuinely care about such individuals when we continue to accept and endorse either their supporting arguments or their behavior. Psychotherapists and sex therapists especially are to blame when they actively encourage an individual to adopt so destructive a lifestyle under the auspices of counseling help.

14

Where Will It End?
A Possible Scenario

There is a despairing theory in health education that says until there is some horrible baseline number of people who have died, the disease doesn't become personal enough to the rest of the community for it to take fundamental changes in behavior seriously.

Dr. Richard Keeling, chairman,
American College Health Association's
Task Force on AIDS

The year is 2030. Most who are now reading this book have died of natural causes. But their children exist in a new world.

Millions of parents have watched their sons and daughters die the agonizing death of AIDS. Millions of teens have watched their parents do the same: thirty-five million Americans have died. Further, American life is unrecognizable by 1990s standards:

- One-half *billion* individual cases of sexually transmitted diseases have been endured.
- Homosexuality, prostitution, and sex outside of marriage are illegal.
- The publishers of pornographic magazines were long ago jailed for crimes against society.
- X and R rated movies, lewd bars, and other sexually explicit activities are banned by law.
- Social dating is strictly regulated by society and parental authority.
- The U.S. health care system is in shambles.

Worldwide the situation is worse:

- 400 million are infected with the HIV virus; 240 million have died.
- Since 1960, *more than ten billion* cases of other sexually transmitted diseases have brought suffering and even death to millions of infants and adults in the world.

- The overall financial costs of the sexual revolution total $50–75 trillion.

Newsreels are now shown in history classrooms with leading athletes, movie stars, and politicians advocating "safe sex," of homosexuals by the hundreds and thousands marching proudly in the streets, and of televised condom ads. These newsreels are used to illustrate a painful lesson of history: how easily society can ignore warning signs that could have prevented tragedy, and the consequences of giving in to powerful special interest groups when public health is at risk.

But now the world economy is in a major depression fueled primarily by national debt and the spiraling costs of the sexual revolution. What this revolution began in the late 1950s has, within a century, destroyed more lives than all previous plagues in recorded human history.

In 2030 no one can quite grasp the irony of the times—times that encouraged the very activity that killed so many millions. The reassuring slogans and promises by leading politicians, social scientists, and sex experts have proved hollow.

Back in the 1990s, there was still a chance for preventing worldwide plague. Unfortunately, few listened; the discipline of abstinence was considered too prudish; standard public health measures were never applied for fear of offending the "civil rights" of certain minority groups, and value-free sex education continued to dominate public education. The end result in 2030: the world is in a morally induced social and political chaos.

Fantasy? Perhaps. Perhaps not. Nevertheless, future generations will look back in disbelief at the sexual behaviors of the last half of the twentieth century. Some will understand the irony of one hundred million AIDS deaths following one hundred million abortions. The generation that murdered tens of millions of unborn human children in various stages of development has, by the same act that created them, proceeded to destroy itself by the tens of millions.

Whatever the outcome, no one will doubt that the sexual revolution of the 1960s wasn't worth it.

Postscript
A Word to Parents

This book has supplied evidence that all of us—parents especially—have a problem. Think about the following illustration revealed by the latest data. Line up two hundred nineteen-year-old single men and women, one hundred of each gender:

- Eighty-seven of the men have already had sexual intercourse.
- Seventy-five of the women have already had sexual intercourse.
- Of the eighty-seven men, half had their first sexual encounter between the ages of eleven and thirteen.
- The average age of having sex was fourteen for boys, fifteen for girls.

So what can we do? The more important question is, "What can *parents* do?" Parents have the ability to exert the most powerful influence on teenage sexual behavior. But they need to have the answers to some basic questions.

Why Do Young People Become Involved Sexually?

By understanding some of the reasons that teens become sexually active, parents can think through appropriate ways to counter such influences. Talking about his own children, one father said, "A child in school today has more sexual temptation than sailors on shore leave." Here are some of the reasons young people get involved sexually.

This chapter is a revised version of a lecture given by John Ankerberg, based in part on the early tapes and lectures of Josh McDowell, most of which were subsequently published in his *Why Wait?*—plus information taken from "The John Ankerberg Show" television programs on (1) "The Playboy Philosophy," (2) "How Safe Is 'Safe Sex' Medically?," (3) "The Transmission of AIDS," and (4) "Planned Parenthood," a program that, as of November 1992, was yet to be aired.

1. *It feels good.* More than 50 percent of the teens surveyed said they get involved sexually simply because they enjoy it.

2. *Peer pressure.* Someone might say, "Well, hasn't peer pressure always been around?" But peer pressure today is different from what parents experienced when they were growing up. The peer pressure then was to not be involved sexually. Now it has been reversed, and a person is expected to be involved sexually. If you're a parent, think back to your own dating days. How hard would it have been for you if the expectation about any given date was that you would become involved sexually?

3. *The media.* The average ten year old sees thousands of acts or alleged acts of sex every year on TV. That means that, by the time a child becomes twenty years old, he has seen tens of thousands of acts of sex on television.

4. *Broken homes.* A child from a two-parent home has twice the encouragement for coping with sexual pressure because he has twice the reinforcement to resist it.

5. *Lack of moral standards.* Young people want direction. In one survey, 67 percent said they wanted to know how to say no to sexual pressure. They want to know what is right and what is wrong. They want to know what is appropriate. Without this, they easily give in to cultural attitudes and peer pressure. Yet at "The John Ankerberg Show" we have talked with Christian teachers in the public schools who have actually been forbidden to teach moral values in the classroom—on threat of dismissal. It is quite a commentary on our times when those whose primary concern is the upholding of personal values—values that all civilized cultures have deemed are important—are threatened with punitive action or labeled as "far right bigots."

6. *Alcohol and drugs.* These break down inhibitions and standards. Many teens have said, "I was under the influence of drugs [or alcohol] and woke up the next morning and realized I was no longer a virgin."

7. *Easy access to birth control.* Concern over the consequences of pregnancy used to be a much greater factor in sexual behavior. Today, the results of sex clinics giving birth control pills to teenagers have been disastrous.

8. *The search for security and self-esteem.* For the male teenager, sex may make him feel that he is a man. For the woman, sex may make her feel loved and desirable. Sex is frequently a search for intimacy, for a feeling of being close to someone and of being able to be "real" around someone. It's a way to be popular or a way to escape loneliness.

9. *The lack of a healthy, biblical understanding of the meaning and purpose of sex.*

In 1 Thessalonians 4 the apostle Paul says, "for you know what instructions we gave you by the authority of the Lord Jesus. It is God's will that you should be sanctified: that you should avoid sexual immorality." When teenagers hear their parents admonish them with "Sex is wrong" or "God says no" or "You are not to have sex before marriage," they may have a negative response. Because of the permissiveness in our culture, parents with moral standards for their children sometimes meet resistance, especially if it is based on religious principles.

Still, behind every negative rule that God gives us, there are always positive principles that God wishes us to know about. For example, God says no because *He wants to protect us* and *He wants to provide the best for us in a mate because He loves us.*

As a parent, I'm constantly giving my daughter Michelle negative commandments: "Don't do this. Don't do that." But I do it because I love her. I don't say no because I want to make life difficult or painful for her. In fact, I know it can be far more painful for her if I give her no rules at all. I already know that when we get outside the limits God has prescribed for us, there is a price to be paid. So my discipline is one of the strongest evidences of my love for her and my commitment to her happiness. Children who may have a difficult time understanding this now will understand it later.

Think of a depressed canary in his cage. He looks out the window at all the birds enjoying life outside and says, "I am trapped in this cage. I can't get out to where the action is and party." So he garners his courage and decides to make a break for it. When he does, at first he thinks, "Now, I'm free. I can do whatever I want." But, instead, he only begins to suffer. He never knew his wings were clipped or that he couldn't fly. He never knew he would be still trapped inside a

Nathan the prophet said, "By doing this, you have made the enemies of the Lord show utter contempt" (2 Samuel 12:14). That is, non-Christians will not take the things of God seriously if Christian young people ignore what God has said and engage in sex outside of marriage.

What Factors Have Studies Shown to Be Successful in Reducing Sexual Involvement Among Teenagers?

1. Statistics show that comprehensive sex education programs are a disaster. So are the "mixed message" programs that make having sex or abstinence morally equal choices. Research shows that only abstinence programs
   - deliver less sexual promiscuity
   - result in fewer teen pregnancies
   - result in fewer abortions
   - cause fewer sexually transmitted diseases
   - cause fewer emotional problems that result from the above
   - produce attitude changes that affect conduct

2. A strong, personal belief, backed by moral conviction that premarital intercourse is usually or always wrong is a vital factor.

3. Adolescents living with both parents have the least permissive views of premarital sex, followed by those living with a parent who has remarried.

4. Teenagers who live in homes where parental discipline is moderately high are twice as likely to avoid premarital intercourse as those whose parents are not strict at all.

5. Teens who report that their parents have moderately strict rules about dating are more likely to abstain from premarital intercourse than those who have no rules or excessive rules.

6. Teens who have parents that are interested and involved in their grades and personal achievements are twice as likely to abstain from sex as those who have parents who do not believe their grades or achievements are important. Not surprisingly, teenagers who attain high academic grades are more likely to abstain from premarital intercourse than those who have lower grades.

7. Teens who look to the future by making plans for higher education

not enough to change my lifestyle. But when AIDS began to spread, that got my attention. I changed my lifestyle and quit sleeping around. I waited until I found the girl of my dreams. Then I married her. After I married her, I found out she had AIDS."

3. God wants to protect us from not being able to discern the difference between love and sex, and God wants to provide a logical basis for our knowing whether we are in love or whether it is just our hormones. Too often sexual enjoyment is mistaken for love, and people get married on the attraction of sex alone. But sex alone will never hold a marriage relationship together because it was never intended to. It was intended to complement a relationship where real love and commitment already exist. Sex is like a rich dessert that complements a fine meal. But if there never is a meal to begin with, eating desserts only will make you sick. Some people say, "Well, it feels like love, so it must be love." But feelings can be terribly deceptive. That is why God has given us a test to see whether or not something is real love or not (see 1 Corinthians 13:4-7).

4. God wants to protect us from having the physical aspect of sex become the dominant part of the relationship. God wants us to truly get to know the other person. Once young people enter into a physical relationship, they may quit communicating. Sex becomes the dominant factor and they never really get to know the other person. The quality of the relationship is reduced to having someone around to satisfy your sexual desires. God also wants to help us protect our virginity. A fifteen-year-old girl said that her girlfriends were pressuring her to have sex. One day she sat them down and said, "Look, just lay off. Any day that I want to, I can become like you. But you can never again become like me." That's true. The greatest gift a man can give to his wife is his purity, his virginity. When you do, and you have sex with that one person that you love and have given yourself to, your mind will remember it, and it will become a bonding experience. It will be something good to remember, and there will be no ghosts of the past.

5. God wants to help Christian young people stay pure so that they can keep their Christian testimony. When David sinned with Bathsheba—and then killed Uriah, her husband, to cover his sin—

Nathan the prophet said, "By doing this, you have made the enemies of the Lord show utter contempt" (2 Samuel 12:14). That is, non-Christians will not take the things of God seriously if Christian young people ignore what God has said and engage in sex outside of marriage.

What Factors Have Studies Shown to Be Successful in Reducing Sexual Involvement Among Teenagers?

1. Statistics show that comprehensive sex education programs are a disaster. So are the "mixed message" programs that make having sex or abstinence morally equal choices. Research shows that only abstinence programs:
   - deliver less sexual promiscuity
   - result in fewer teen pregnancies
   - result in fewer abortions
   - cause fewer sexually transmitted diseases
   - cause fewer emotional problems that result from the above
   - produce attitude changes that affect conduct

2. A strong, personal belief, backed by moral conviction that premarital intercourse is usually or always wrong is a vital factor.

3. Adolescents living with both parents have the least permissive views of premarital sex, followed by those living with a parent who has remarried.

4. Teenagers who live in homes where parental discipline is moderately high are twice as likely to avoid premarital intercourse as those whose parents are not strict at all.

5. Teens who report that their parents have moderately strict rules about dating are more likely to abstain from premarital intercourse than those who have no rules or excessive rules.

6. Teens who have parents that are interested and involved in their grades and personal achievements are twice as likely to abstain from sex as those who have parents who do not believe their grades or achievements are important. Not surprisingly, teenagers who attain high academic grades are more likely to abstain from premarital intercourse than those who have lower grades.

7. Teens who look to the future by making plans for higher education

and who regard marriage highly are more likely to abstain from premarital intercourse than those who don't.

8. Teens who delay dating and avoid steady dating are more likely to abstain from premarital intercourse.

9. Teens who report that religion is important to them are more likely to abstain than teenagers who say religion is not important.

10. Teenage girls who report a close mother/daughter relationship are more likely to abstain from sex than those who do not have this relationship.

How Can Parents Help Their Kids Cope with Sexual Pressures Today?

Don't accept the myth that says, "Our kids are hopeless, they will do it anyway." Teenagers may say, "Everywhere I turn, I see sex. Sex education, Planned Parenthood, television, movies, and my friends all tell me the same message: 'Now is the time to be involved sexually.' The philosophy everywhere is that since we are going to be sexually involved anyway, give us birth control and show us how to use condoms."

Parents need to help their children see the error of this approach by applying this same reasoning to drugs—another powerful experience. This nation should be grateful that Planned Parenthood is not in charge of our drug program. Just think what things would be like if our drug programs had the following philosophy: "I don't care what you say. Most kids are going to take drugs regardless, and there's nothing we can do about it. So we need to make it safe. We need to have drug clinics at our schools; we need to pass out clean needles, and we must give our children safe places to get high and come down."

When educators say our kids are going to do it anyway, what they're really implying is that our kids don't have the character or cannot develop the character to say no. What an insult to our children! They'll say, "Look at sexual involvement today. Look how high it is. That's proof." But isn't that admitting what everyone really knows— that there was a time when kids really weren't sexually involved? The truth is that our kids are not helpless. They can say no with a little encouragement. But if we assume they have the morals of an alley cat, should we be surprised at the outcome?

Don't compromise by saying it's OK to say no. It's not just OK, it's *right* to say no. Today especially, it's the smartest and wisest thing to do.

How can parents help children verbalize the right attitudes when they are under pressure from their friends to have sex? One way is to teach your children effective responses. These can be modified for different situations. The point is to help your kids make their feelings clear up front without unnecessarily damaging a potential friendship. Of course, if Christian young people restrict their dating to those who are also committed to virginity, this approach is unnecessary.

But here is one approach. The first and second time your children are pressured to have sex, they should emphatically say no. The third time, they should share their feelings. For example, they should say to their friend, "How do you think this makes me feel? It makes me feel that all you think about is that I'm a sex object. I'm not. I'm a person. But all you seem to care about is sex. Do you care about what I think or what I feel? Or do you just care about your own desires?"

The fourth time, if they have said no and shared their feelings, and they're still pressured to have sex, then they should walk away from that person, because he or she is not a true friend. Your child is better than that and deserves more from life than what that person has to offer.

But what do you do if, for whatever reason, your kids find it difficult to be so direct with a negative answer? Some people may find it difficult to say no. For a man it may be seen as a threat to his manliness or his self-esteem. If a girl pressures him to have sex, he feels it is his manly "duty" to do so. Or, if a girl says no to a man's sexual pressure, the guy may think he has to push her even more to "prove" his manhood. Or, for a woman, if someone says no to her sexual pressure, she may think, "Well, what's wrong with me. Aren't I desirable?" To handle this situation, teach your children to try a reinforcement approach that keeps communication clear and open. Begin with a positive reinforcement, then insert the negative, and then close with another positive reinforcement.

For example, say a guy pressures a girl to come over to study with him. He calls and says, "I'd really like for you to come on over. My parents are gone, and we can study together." But she knows he has other things on his mind than history books. What can she say? She should start with the positive. "Jim, I'd love to study with you. You're a lot of fun to study with." That's a positive statement. Then put in the negative: "But I don't think it would be a good idea for me to come and study with you when your parents are away." Now the positive: "But I think the library is open. Why don't we go there to study?"

If your children learn to develop an overall positive approach that still permits them to avoid compromising situations, it can help them to say no.

Other Ways to Help Your Children

Have them write out their convictions about sex. What do they believe? What standard will they live their lives according to? Have your children do this with Christ, God, the Bible, sin, sex, family, drugs, marriage, personal dating standards, and so on. This will help them formulate their convictions. Parents should help their kids along the way. It is a great time for family sharing of the important issues in life—issues that can dramatically affect the quality of their future.

Encourage your children to set their standards before they date. Kids must know their convictions before they set their standards and know why they must set their standards before they date. With all the pressure from TV, movies, books, and music, it's best to start by having them think through their convictions so they can set their standards before becoming involved in a dating relationship.

Parents always model standards for their children. Don't expect your young people to have standards stricter than your own. How do you live? How do you talk? What do you watch? What do you read? How do you treat your wife/husband? Your children are picking up on all of it. If you want your kids to respond in the right direction, they have to see these standards in your own life. If children don't see them in parents' lives, then parents shouldn't expect to see them in their children's lives. Parenting isn't just rearing children and enjoying them; it's a responsibility to mold their character and provide them with the gift of a positive start in life.

Have young people plan their dates. Many young people say, "It was on those dates when we had nothing to do that we got sexually involved." So parents should ask certain questions: "Where are you going on your date? What are you going to do? When will you be back? Who will you be with?"

Parents might think, "Kids won't go for that." But you're wrong. They will go for it. It's very interesting to see how many teenagers will use their parents as the excuse they need to respond to sexual peer pressure: "I can't do that because I have to be in by 10:00," or, "I can't go to that kind of party because my parents wouldn't approve." Kids know what is right and wrong more, perhaps, than we give them credit for, and often they are looking for ways to avoid situations they know they can't handle. When parents have communicated their standards to the kids and have stood firm, such parental concern gives the kids a legitimate chance to make wise decisions under peer pressure.

It's good for teens to briefly pray together on a date. But encourage them not to hold hands or pray about their negative feelings. (For example, "Oh, Lord, I feel so lonely tonight. I wish that somebody would really love me.") Be cautious about having kids pray together or read the Bible together for a long time, because it may lead to physical intimacy. But a brief prayer, committing their goals and time together, helps. They can express their love to the Lord and their desire to please and obey Him on their date.

Teach your children to communicate their standards up front to those they date. This is crucial. At the start, kids need to communicate clearly things such as: "I don't want to kiss or pet. I want to get to know you as a person. I want to find out if we can be good friends."

How Far Should Kids Go in Dating?

Parents can help their children by having them think of someone they really respect. "What would that person think if he (or she) saw what you were doing? What if Jesus Christ were sitting right there next to you. What would He think? Isn't He the one we should be concerned about?" Parents should help their children understand that the other person's sexual life belongs to God and his/her future marriage partner, not to them. A man should treat a woman on a date the same way he would want any other man to treat the woman he will someday marry. Teach them not to take something that doesn't belong to them. Every young boy should remember that the girl he is with will someday be somebody's wife. If he is pressuring her to have sex, then he is taking something that ultimately does not belong to him.

If teenagers "fall in love," the pressures may increase, because it is at this point especially that their values are tested. Help them to see that, if they really are "in love," then what a perfect opportunity to prove it by living out the standards of love with the one they care for so deeply. In other words, if they have abstained from sex with those they didn't love, how much more should they do so for the one they do love. When you meet "Mr. Right," or the dream girl of your life, stick to your standards.

Explain to your teenagers that they have gone too far when they can no longer make an intelligent and responsible decision and act that decision out—that is, the moment they have become aroused and begin to act that out, they have lost their freedom. An aroused hormone has no conscience. When they realize that the only way they can satisfy their aroused hormones is to go outside the limits God has placed, then they are on dangerous ground and must react immediately.

How Can Parents Encourage the Right Kind of Peer Pressure upon their Children?

How can parents make sure the right kind of friends are involved with their child? First, look around at the different kinds of kids. Are there good kids in sports, music, church, science clubs, arts and crafts? Then encourage your kids to participate in those areas. Soon you'll find out that your kids will be hanging around with those kids, and they'll have quality friends. Pray that God will give you ideas and direct you so that you surround your kids with positive peer pressure.

What Can Parents Do to Reduce Teen Sexual Involvement?

Don't let your kids date too early. One guideline here is to tell your kids they're not old enough to date until they can say no to sexual pressure and follow through on it. Children must show by their character and lifestyle that they can say no and mean it. If they can't, they shouldn't date. Explain to them that you wouldn't be a loving parent if you didn't take such an approach. Remember, ts who delay starting to date and avoid steady dating are more likely to abstain from premarital intercourse than those who do not. Of those girls who begin dating at:

- Twelve years of age, 90 percent will have sexual intercourse before marriage
- Thirteen years of age: 58 percent
- Fourteen years of age: 50 percent
- Fifteen years of age: 40 percent
- Sixteen years of age: 19 percent
- Seventeen years of age: 15 percent

Kids aren't old enough to date until they show maturity. What is maturity? Maturity is the ability to delay immediate gratification. Kids may respond with, "Well, how will you know I've reached that point?" Tell them that their behavior and the choices they make in other areas will tell you. Look how they handle eating ice cream, or watching a movie or a television program, or how they talk to their friends on the phone or buy a certain record or clothing. Can they postpone immediate physical gratification? If they can, they are becoming mature. Any child can give in to sexual desires, but it takes a mature teen to say no, to mean it, and to wait.

Have the young people in your church youth group (or other group) hold each other accountable to staying pure. This really works. It encourages each person to maintain the standards they agreed upon. It's a reason for them to stay pure, and it teaches them social and personal accountability.

Church attendance is important. Research shows that a child who goes to church just once a week will be less involved sexually. That's a great influence on a child.

Have proper morals taught in sex education. No one can teach morally neutral sex education. Sex always involves two people; it is a social act. So how can anyone teach sex without also teaching character? We've got to put sex in a moral context. Character is the basis of how people learn to relate to others and to care for people. That is why personal character must be taught in sex education. And it is also why the source of morals from sex education must come from the parents.

Kids want to know that there are limits. If the statistics show that 50 percent of the men who are now nineteen had their first sexual experience between the time of eleven and thirteen, then parents can't wait for the big sex talk until fourteen—it has to come earlier. How early? A good rule of thumb is this: little questions deserve little answers; big questions deserve big answers; frank questions deserve frank answers. Give them just enough to answer their questions at their age level.

How Can Parents Help Young People Handle the "Pressure Lines"?

There are many ways to provide your children with proper responses to sexual pressure. Here are some responses you could rehearse with them.

Line: "I love you so much."
Response: "Is sex love?"

Line: "Well, if you love me, you'll let me."
Response: "If you did love me, you wouldn't persist in pressuring me to do something I don't want to do and that isn't good for either of us."

Line: "Everyone else is doing it."
Response: "That's OK. I don't want to be like everyone else, and I certainly don't what everybody else has—STDs, guilt, divorce, or AIDS. I don't want that."

Line: "Well, all the other girls are doing it."
Response: "So, date them. I'm not like them."

Line: "You're not a man if you don't!"
Response: "What would you know about being a man?"

Line: "I would never get married unless I know we are sexually compatible."
Response: "Then I guess we aren't."

Line: "Come on, it feels so good."
Response: "So does doing drugs; that's not the issue."

Remember, the research shows that for all teenagers, the number one resource they would like to have for information about sex is mom and dad.

The time a child doesn't want to get information about sex from mom and dad may be when he's just engaged in sex. Parental contact usually adds to the guilt, so this is the one time the child doesn't want mom and dad involved. But this is exactly when parents need to extend the grace of God to their kids. If through the death of Jesus Christ on the cross God cannot deal with sexual sin, then He can't deal with any sin. After the fact, we need to be ready to extend forgiveness, to help our children get up and get back on the right road.

1. *Admit your sin.* Somebody may say, "Can I become a virgin again if I admitted sin?" No. You can only give up your virginity once, but spiritually you can become a virgin again in your mind. You can have your mind cleansed. So number one, admit that it's sin.

2. *Confess it.* First John 1:9 says, "If we confess our sins, He is faithful and just to forgive us our sins and to cleanse us from all unrighteousness."

3. *Acknowledge God's forgiveness and forgive yourself.* Anytime you don't forgive yourself you're saying two things: first, you have a higher standard than God, and, second, Jesus Christ's death on the cross was not sufficient for your sin.

4. *Show fruits of repentance.* This may include breaking off with the person that you committed that sin with or saying, "I won't go to that kind of party again. I won't see that kind of a movie or listen to that kind of a record again."

5. *Don't feel condemned, just convicted.* The Holy Spirit points out when something is wrong and convicts us not to do it again. But when He does this, He points us to Christ for forgiveness. When God says, "Don't commit sexual immorality," He says it because He loves us and wants to protect us. It is Satan who condemns and attempts to foster the guilt and self-hatred that can be so destructive, especially to sensitive teenagers.

Children are a precious gift from the Lord and a terrible thing to waste. "Behold, children are a gift of the Lord; the fruit of the womb is a reward" (Psalm 127:3). Although formative years can be wasted, it is never too late to begin to educate your children in godliness.

Parents are privileged to have one of the most enjoyable and rewarding experiences in all of life: to raise their children so that they become wise and godly young men and women—people whose principal goal in life is to serve and honor Jesus Christ, no matter what vocation they choose. "Train up a child in the way he should go, even when he is old he will not depart from it" (Proverbs 22:6).

What If My Kids Are Christian?

Parents of kids who have professed faith in Christ before or during their teen years might feel a false sense of security regarding their kid's possible involvement in teen sexual activity. However, the "Why Wait?" Church Teen Sexuality Survey (Josh McDowell Ministry) indicates otherwise.

- By eighteen, 43 percent of churched youth have had sexual intercourse.
- By eighteen, 65 percent of churched youth have had sexual contact, from fondling to intercourse.
- More than one-third (36 percent) of churched teens felt that intercourse between two consenting individuals was morally acceptable.
- Sexual contact was much less likely among those teens who had a close relationship with their father.
- Teens surveyed that have not had a "born again" experience were more than twice as likely to have had sexual relations.
- Those youth who spent a large amount of time with popular media were much more likely to have sexual contact.
- Nearly three out of five teens who reported seeing an R-rated movie had had sexual contact.
- the major sources of information about sex were friends (38 percent), movies (26 percent), parents (23 percent), television (22 percent), and schools (23 percent).

Teen sex among churched youth is a significant problem. Parents of Christian teenagers should not assume that their kids will abstain from sex without their loving and firm supervision, help, and support.

Appendix 1

Two Views of Sex:

Those who—with good motives to be sure—want to turn this country into a sexual wasteland—the pornographers, homosexual lobbyists, and son one—base their attitudes toward sex on an anti-Christian philosophy. In the chart below, the differences between the Christian and the secular (materialist) view of sexuality are illustrated:

THE CHRISTIAN/BIBLICAL VIEW OF SEX	THE LIBERAL SECULAR/ HUMANIST VIEW OF SEX
Sex is a precious gift of God.	Sex is a biological, animal function without divine aspect or intent.
The sexual act and its results are to be protected by restriction to marriage.	The sexual act has no restrictions among *consenting* parties, including all varieties of heterosexual acts, homosexual acts, sadomasochistic sex, sex between adults and children, sex between adults and animals, whatever a person chooses.
The purpose of sex is the expression of committed love, for bonding in marriage, procreation, and physical-emotional pleasure.	The purpose of sex is primarily sensualistic pleasure without *necessary* connections to marriage or commitment.

THE CHRISTIAN/BIBLICAL VIEW OF SEX
(CONTINUED)

The sexual act itself is a physical analogy and parallel to the nature of God and what He accomplished spiritually in the incarnation and atonement in Christ.

The Christian view of sex and marriage functions to protect children and restrict divorce.

The Christian view of sex offers a genuine solution: Those who follow the Christian view of sex prohibit the possibility of unwanted pregnancy, abortion, guilt, AIDS, and other sexually transmitted diseases. (Those who follow the Christian view of sex will not die from the sexual act.)

THE LIBERAL SECULAR/ HUMANIST VIEW OF SEX
(CONTINUED)

The nature of sex is primarily a natural (animal) function destitute of any theological implication.

The liberal view of sex frequently leads to divorce and functions to injure children emotionally.

The secular view continues the tragedy: Those who engage in sex freely run high risks of severe physical or emotional consequences. They risk AIDS and other sexually transmitted diseases and are now transmitting them to others throughout the population.

Appendix 2

Statistics About Sexual Behavior

(Excerpted from *Psychological Reports*, vol. 64 [1989], 1171–74; used with permission of The Family Research Institute, Washington, D.C.)

TABLE 1

CLAIMED EXPOSURE TO INDIVIDUAL AND PUBLIC HEALTH RISKS: PERCENT EVER REPORTING EXPERIENCE

Activity/Behavior	Sex	Hetro-sexual	Bi-sexual	Homo-sexual	Relative Risk†	Cluster
n	M	1,261	36	41		
	F	1,990	42	24		
Sadomasochism	M	5	28	37	6.6	C
	F	4	21	8	4.1	C
Bondage	M	10	25	32	2.9	C
	F	7	44	17	5.0	C
Fist in anus ("handballing")	M	2	33	42	18.8	C
	F	1	33	8	24.7	C
Urination ("golden shower")	M	4	14	29	5.8	C
	F	2	17	‡	4.6	C
Defecation ("scat")	M	1	‡	17	10.1	C
	F	1	2	‡	1.7*	C
Enemas	M	2	11	12	4.9	C
	F	1	15	‡	8.4	C
Sex with animals	M	3	19	15	6.4	C
	F	1	15	‡	11.0	C
Paying for sex	M	34	28	34	.9*	A
	F	‡	7	‡	12.8	A
Paid for sex	M	5	22	23	4.5	A
	F	3	29	9	11.2	A
Threesomes, orgies, or group sex	M	22	61	88	3.4	A,C
	F	7	71	25	8.0	A,C
Sex in gay bath	M	1	42	68	57.6	A,B
	F	‡	10	‡	15.9	A,B
Sex in peep show or booth	M	5	38	50	8.8	B
	F	1	29	‡	13.8	B
Sex in public restroom	M	6	28	66	7.2	B
	F	2	24	9	8.2	B

TABLE 1

(CONTINUED)

CLAIMED EXPOSURE TO INDIVIDUAL AND PUBLIC HEALTH RISKS:
PERCENT EVER REPORTING EXPERIENCE

Activity/Behavior	Sex	Hetro-sexual	Bi-sexual	Homo-sexual	Relative Risk†	Cluster
n	M	1,243	36	42		
	F	1,932	40	23		
Heterosexual kiss	M	97	100	88	1.0*	C
	F	100	98	100	1.0*	C
Oral genital sex on male	M	4	92	100	24.0	C
	F	75	90	57	1.0*	C
Oral genital sex on female	M	79	86	31	.7	C
	F	1	90	96	92.0*	C
Perform anal sex on male	M	2	75	93	42.3	C
	F	19	50	17	2.0	C
Perform anal sex on female	M	36	33	2	.4	C
	F	‡	28	48	337.4	C
Ever in hetero orgy	M	12	17	‡	.6*	A,C
	F	4	33	‡	5.2	A,C
Ever in bisexual orgy	M	1	25	2	11.5*	A,C
	F	1	35	17	27.1	A,C
Ever in homosexual orgy	M	‡	39	67	685.8*	A,C
	F	‡	10	9	64.1	A,C
n	M	1,345	‡ 39	4167		
	F	2,094	44	25		
Ever had STD	M	30	52	85	2.3	D
	F	24	43	18	1.5*	D
Oral anal contact	M	25	68	92	3.3	C
	F	32	61	53	1.8	C
Smoke tobacco	M	37	28	56	1.1*	D
	F	37	49	40	1.2*	D
Regular high on any drug	M	37	36	46	1.1*	D
	F	20	64	32	2.4	D
Ever raped	M	3	13	12	4.2	A
	F	15	62	32	3.4	A

*Groups not significantly different at $p < .05$. For other tested comparisons $p < .001$ by x^2.
†Relative risk in the ratio of percentages of homosexual/bisexual vs heterosexual who claimed the experience/behavior.
‡0 or $< 0.5\%$.

TABLE 2

CLAIMED NUMBERS OF SEXUAL PARTNERS AND DURATION OF SEXUAL RELATIONSHIPS:
MEDIAN FREQUENCIES AND LENGTHS

Activity/Behavior	Sex	Hetero-sexual	Bi-sexual	Homo-sexual
n	M	1,345	39	41
	F	2,094	44	25
Mdn No. different homosexual partners last year	M	†	3	10
	F	†	1	1
Mdn No. different lifetime homosexual partners	M	†	10	100
	F	†	3	4
Mdn No. different heterosexual partners last year	M	1	2	†
	F	1	2	†
Mdn No. different lifetime heterosexual partners	M	8	6	2
	F	3	10	3
Mdn No. different lifetime sexual partners	M	8	16	101
	F	3	13	7
Mdn No. longest completely faithful heterosexual relationship	M	5 – 10 yr.	<2 yr.	<1 yr.
	F	5 – 10 yr.	<3 mo.	<1 yr.
Mdn No. longest completely faithful homosexual relationship	M	†	<3 mo.	<1 yr.
	F	†	<1 yr.	3 – 4 yr.

†0 or <0.5%.

TABLE 3

INDICES OF SOCIAL DISRUPTION/COHESION: PERCENT EVER REPORTING EXPERIENCE

Activity/Behavior	Sex	Hetero-sexual	Bi-sexual	Homo-sexual	Relative	p
n	M	1,345	39	41		
	F	2,094	44	25		
Always/usually wear seat belt	M	31	41	29	1.1*	
	F	33	33	17	.8*	
Traffic ticket in past 5 yr.	M	53	69	44	1.1*	
	F	33	46	54	1.5	<0.04
Traffic accident in past 5 yr.	M	38	38	41	1.0*	
	F	29	57	27	1.7	<0.005
Ever drive carelessly	M	76	74	70	1.0*	
	F	69	81	78	1.2*	
Contemplated suicide	M	27	51	41	1.7	<.001
	F	34	62	50	1.7*	<.001
Attempted suicide	M	5	15	22	1.7	<.001
	F	10	24	17	2.2*	<.005
Attempted suicide	M	3	35	‡	.4*	
	F	20	31	30	1.5	<.04
Made obscene phone call	M	8	8	21	1.8	<.04
	F	3	13	9	1.5	<.001
Had sex in front others	M	24	59	71	2.7	<.001
	F	7	56	17	5.9	<.001
Had sex in front others	M	17	40	44	2.5	<.001
	F	5	37	9	5.5	<.001

TABLE 3

(CONTINUED)

INDICES OF SOCIAL DISRUPTION/COHESION: PERCENT EVER REPORTING EXPERIENCE

Activity/Behavior	Sex	Hetero-sexual	Bi-sexual	Homo-sexual	Relative	p
Had sex in Jail	M	1	‡	10	5.2	<.02
	F	‡	10	‡	8.8	<.02
Ever had sex to infect others	M	7	14	‡	3.1	<.001
	F	1	14	‡	3.1	<.001
No. infected/100 of that	M	~5[a]	12	12		
orientation	F	~4[a]	146	5	3.1	<.001
n	M	1,337	39	42		
	F	2,076	44	25		
Physical fight last year	M	16	11	17	.9*	
	F	6	21	17	3.3	<.001
Ever tried to/did kill another	M	12	8	10	.8*	
	F	1	14	4	7.8	<.001
Ever in trouble in school	M	79	71	56	.8*	<.02
	F	48	70	80	1.7	<.001
Ever arrested for nonsexual crime	M	22	8	24	.7	
	F	5	18	12	3.2	<.001
Ever arrested for sexual crime	M	1	3	7	5.1	<.001
	F	‡	7	‡	10.9	<.001
Ever convicted of nonsexual crime	M	11	8	10	.8*	
	F	2	5	8	3.0*	<.001
Ever convicted of sexual crime	M	1	3	2	2.5*	
	F	‡	5	‡	2.5	<.02
Ever jailed for crime	M	13	13	17	.9*	
	F	3	14	8	3.9	<.01
Ever homosexual sex in jail	M	1	‡	5	5.0*	
	F	‡	9	‡	8.7	<.005
Ever not caught for crime	M	34	31	37	1.0*	
	F	15	34	24	2.0	<.005
Ever not caught for sex crime	M	7	36	24	4.5	<.03
	F	1	14	12	22.5	<.001
Ever shoplift	M	52	46	55	1.0*	
	F	36	74	76	2.1	<.001
Ever cheat on income tax	M	15	26	27	1.8	<.02
	F	8	11	12	1.4*	
Ever married	M	72	46	19	.4	<.001
	F	82	51	40	.6	<.001
Currently in first marriage	M	46	21	5	.3	<.001
	F	51	16	4	.2	<.001
Cheated in first marriage	M	31	65	100	2.5	<.001
	F	20	76	50	.2	<.001
Cheated in first subsequent	M	24	50	50	2.1*	
marriage	F	19	67	33	2.9	<.005

*Groups not significantly different a $p < 0.05$. For other tested comparisons $p < 0.001$ by x^2.

†Relative risk in the ratio of percentages of homosexuals/bisexuals vs heterosexuals who claimed the experience/ behavior.

‡0 or <0.5%.

Appendix 3
Is AIDS a Divine Judgment on Sexual Promiscuity?

According to J. Gordon Melton's Institute for the Study of American Religion, almost no one believes that AIDS is God's punishment for immoral behavior. Melton reviewed the policies of some fifty groups, including Protestants, Catholics, Jews, Muslims, and Buddhists, for a new book entitled *The Churches Speak on AIDS*. His conclusion was that almost no one believes that AIDS is an expression of God's wrath. "Almost universally, whether liberal or conservative, the groups are saying that it's *bad theology* to say this is a judgment of God." Melton concludes, "Almost no one today believes God singles out individuals or groups for special punishment in their lifetimes. God doesn't work like that."[1]

On the other hand, Romans 1 states that "the wrath of God is revealed from heaven against all ungodliness and unrighteousness of men, who suppress the truth in unrighteousness."[1] (v. 18 NASB) God's wrath against human sin is consistently revealed throughout the Old Testament and in the book of Revelation. To say that God *never* visits individuals or groups of people with divine judgment for sin is false.

The question is, "In what sense is AIDS a divine judgment?" We believe that AIDS is more a consquence of sinful lifestyle and hence what is properly termed an *indirect* rather than a *direct* judgment of God. In other words, God made men and women in such a manner that there are unavoidable consequences to sin. As Margaret Clarkson writes,

> It is important, however, to distinguish between suffering as judgment for sin and suffering as the consequences of sin. Implicating God's judgment against sin in general is the simple law of cause and effect:

sin gives rise to consequences for those who indulge in it. Just as it is with the [penal] laws of our country, if we transgress against God's natural, moral or spiritual laws, we will suffer the inevitable consequences. God's judgment is set against sin itself rather than against the sinner. If we sin willfully and persistently, we invite the consequences that must follow sin, and this will involve suffering.[2]

Thus, the Bible teaches that it is possible to suffer either God's direct punishment for sin or sin's inescapable consequences. When God's righteous judgment falls upon sin, people suffer the natural results. That is why God says, "Do not be deceived, God is not mocked; for whatever a man sows this he will also reap" (Galatians 6:7 NASB).

So, whether we think AIDS is a direct or indirect judgment upon sin, it is still proof that there are consequences to violating God's laws. God, of course, still loves the sinner and desires that those who are unrepentant will turn to Him for forgiveness of sin. Indeed, this is frequently the case when people suffer for their sins—life becomes so miserable that they do indeed turn to God and cry out for His mercy and salvation.

AIDS is primarily the result of sexual sin, whether homosexual or heterosexual. So the real question is, "Does God judge sin?" Biblically, the answer is yes.

Consider several examples. During the Flood of Noah's day God judged the sin of the world, which at that time was violence and wickedness (Genesis 6:11–13). God condemned the Canaanites for a wide variety of evil practices, including rampant sexual immorality (Deuteronomy 18:9–13; Leviticus 20:22–23). He also judged the E-gyptians, the Jews, and many other cultures (e.g., Jeremiah 44–52).

Thus, God judges sexual sins: "The Lord will punish men for all such sins" (1 Thessalonians 4:6). For example, God destroyed Sodom and Gomorrah; the primary sin of those towns was sodomy (Genesis 19). In fact, God has never ceased judging men or nations (Romans 1:18; Galatians 6:7), nor will He, as the book of Revelation so powerfully demonstrates (chaps. 9–18).

How can anyone say with certainty, then, that AIDS is not in some sense a divine judgment upon sin? But many do argue in this manner, and their passion has convinced many others.

Wendell Hoffman and Stanley Grenz comment, "As a society, we are now reaping the consequences of the attitudes we have developed over the last several decades. There *is* an undeniable connection between societal sin and the spread of AIDS."[3] Hoffman and Grenz also note the unavoidable conclusion that AIDS constitutes a divine judgment.[4] This conclusion derives from several facts.

First, AIDS is a powerful reminder of the relationship between acts and consequences. Second, AIDS is a judgment upon the privatization of morality. (This is the idea that whatever is done between consenting adults is solely and entirely a private matter with no social repercussions.) AIDS forces us to realize that a clear relationship exists between an individual's "private" acts and the public good. Thus, "No people can allow God's norms to be ignored or eroded and expect to suffer no ill consequences."[5] Third, AIDS may also be seen as a judgment upon the callousness of the church in its treatment of sexual offenders such as homosexuals and prostitutes. "To the extent that our unwillingness to become 'community' to persons whose lifestyles we see as abhorrent has contributed to their fleeing to unwholesome communities for fellowship, we contributed to the spread of the epidemic."[6] In other words, "to what degree are homosexually oriented persons driven to the gay community, even to impersonal sex practices and promiscuity, because they are unable to find community within the wider society and more specifically, within our churches? To what extent have we as Christians been guilty of sinning against persons with a homosexual orientation because of our failure to show love and to offer them the true fellowship they are seeking?"[7] The church must show both compassion and mercy on the one hand and exercise a call for repentance to the wider society on the other.

What most people in modern America apparently do not understand is the specific reasons that God treats the sex act seriously. If they understood some of these reasons, they might have a better grasp of why, at some point, judgment becomes necessary.

The first reason God treats the sex act seriously is because, having created us in His own image, He knows the consequences of illicit sexual activity—physical, psychological, and spiritual. Some of these have been outlined in this book, but they are far from the whole story. In essence, we were not created to be able to withstand sexual immorality without suffering consequences. Sexual immorality not only leads to such things as divorce, unwanted pregnancy, abortion, AIDS and other STDs, infertility, guilt, and other serious problems, it also leads to estrangement from God. It separates us from the best that God has for us physically, emotionally, and spiritually.

The sex act is meant to be an expression of the deep love two people hold for one another; to share that essence with others indiscriminately is to profane the relationship of love that it symbolizes. Most who think about it will acknowledge that intercourse is far more than just a physical act. It also has deep emotional and even spiritual undercurrents. In fact, we would say that sex is equally or primarily an emotional/spiritual act before it is a physical act. That is why to treat it as anything less than something holy is to profane it. God intended it to be holy, and that is how it is treated in the Bible.

Perhaps the clearest illustration of the sanctity of the sex act is to understand how it parallels the relationship of Jesus Christ to His church. The Bible itself parallels sexual intercourse with Christ and the church. In Ephesians 5:31–32 we read, "For this reason a man will leave his father and mother and be united to his wife, and the two will become one flesh. This is a profound mystery—but I am talking about Christ and the church" (see 1 Corinthians 6:15–18). Thus, consider the parallel between the sexual act in marriage and what God has done in Christ for His church. A man and a woman will leave their families, come together socially, and before the world make a public declaration of their love for each other at the marriage ceremony. Afterward, a man goes into a woman, and there is joy, unity, and eventually new life. Here we see the parallel to what God has done in the incarnation. Jesus left his "family" (the Father and Spirit) and came to earth to make a public declaration of His love for mankind at the cross. When a person receives Christ, Christ goes into that person, there is joy and unity and a new spiritual birth. Perhaps one reason God treats the sexual act so seriously is because He intended it as an illustration of His own love for mankind. Again, to profane the sexual act is to profane that which it represents.

Some argue that denying AIDS as a punishment from God is part of the thinking that helps perpetuate sexual sin and the diseases it causes. Only when people really believe that God judges sin will they be willing to consider change. Otherwise, change will be forced on them.

Depending on the severity of the sinful conditions, divine judgment may be either complete and retributive (e.g., Noah's Flood, Sodom and Gomorrah; Genesis 6, 19) or partial and remedial (e.g., Nineveh, the Babylonian Captivity). AIDS seems to be a mixture of both. Thankfully, the disease does not end life immediately. But it does send a strong message about the importance of changing behavior. Perhaps that is why the homosexual community has changed its behavior at all. One must ask the question, Would their behavior have changed without a tragedy of sufficient proportions to get their attention? The same reasoning holds true for the sins of the heterosexual community. By asserting that AIDS is not in some sense God's judgment or wrath upon human sin, one may be downplaying God's holiness as well as human responsibility.

Others have argued that AIDS cannot be a divine judgment because there are so many innocent victims, such as hemophiliacs and children. But the fact that innocent victims exist is not a logical argument against AIDS as a divine judgment. Unfortunately, innocent victims always suffer whenever there is judgment. In fact, it could not be otherwise. Consider the illustration of Daniel. Daniel and a godly remnant within Israel were taken captive to Babylon; both the righteous and innocent suffered for the evil deeds of the majority of the nation.

In the same manner an innocent woman, by virtue of being a wife, must of necessity suffer the consequences of her husband's alcoholism or criminal activity—so innocent individuals in an evil society likewise suffer the judgment upon that society. Just as the family is a unit wherein the whole suffers for the sins of one member, society is also a unit. There are many innocent victims of drug abuse and drunk driving.

Without consequences to evil, evil would flourish all the more. With the consequences of AIDS, the principle is the same—God exalts His righteous character in the midst of human sin and in love strikes out in judgment to remove evil. It cannot be doubted that the end result of the AIDS epidemic will force a return to monogamy and godly sexuality. In the process, the great tragedies produced by the "sexual revolution" will be curtailed.

In spite of all this, it is important to remember that, whenever God does judge, His mercy is also operative. This, too, can be seen in the history of His dealings with the Jewish nation in the Old Testament. Though Daniel and his three friends suffered exile, they had such an influence in the court of Nebuchadnezzar that the entire Jewish Diaspora were granted special safeguards.

There is little doubt that AIDS is God's judgment upon sexual immorality. Whether homosexual or heterosexual, the consequences of such behavior over the past thirty years have been appalling. Literally tens of millions of lives have been ruined by sexual promiscuity. Would we expect God to sit back and do nothing while millions more are destroyed?

Nineveh finally repented at the preaching of Jonah and was spared judgment. Israel, on the other hand, was warned by God through the prophets to change her ways; because she did not, captivity fell upon the nation. But this judgment was successful in that it eradicated the rampant idolatry and other evils that had been practiced to that point and changed the national conscience from that time onward. Hopefully AIDS will do the same.

God loves us and desires His best for us. That is why He has told us how to live—what to do and what not to do. If we do what He tells us, our lives will be blessed. If we disobey His commands, we will suffer the natural results.

The Bible teaches that it is God's will that the sexual act be reserved for a committed lifelong relationship between a man and a woman in marriage. Not once does the Bible say that sexual intercourse is permitted outside of marriage. That is why the thrust of human history and in particular the last half of the twentieth century has proven the importance and legitimacy of the Christian view of sex. When God says that sex is to be reserved for marriage, because He made us we can trust Him that He knows what is best (Matthew 15:19; Mark 7:21; Acts 15:20, 29; 21:25; Romans 13:13; 1 Corinthians 5:1; 6:13, 18; 10:8; Galatians 5:19; Ephesians 5:3; Colossians 3:5; 1 Thessalonians 4:3; Jude 7; Revelation 2:4, 20; 9:21).

Notes

Note: The authors express their gratitude to Josh McDowell for his *Research Almanac and Statistical Digest* (San Bernadino, Calif.: Here's Life, 1991), which provided approximately 5 percent of the citations in this book.

CHAPTER 1

1. *Phoenix Gazette*, 20 August 1983.
2. In Josh McDowell, *The Myths of Sex Education* (San Bernardino, Calif.: Here's Life, 1990); cf. *Los Angeles Times,* 19 February 1990, 8.
3. *Parade*, 18 December 1988, 16.
4. *People*, 13 April 1987.
5. Patricia Hersch, "Sexually Transmitted Diseases Are Ravaging Our Children: Teen Epidemic," *American Health*, May 1991; cf., *USA Today,* 8 November 1990, 1a.
6. McDowell, *The Myths of Sex Education*, 9.
7. Hersch, "Sexually Transmitted Diseases," 44.
8. Sam Gitchel and Lorri Foster, *Let's Talk About Sex* (Fresno, Calif.: Planned Parenthood of Central California, n.d.), 5
9. Dinah Richard, *Has Sex Education Failed Our Teenagers? A Research Report* (Pomona, Calif.: Focus on the Family, 1990), 42.
10. William J. Bennett, "Sex and the Education of Our Children," U.S. Department of Education, 22 January 1987; transcript of talk at the National School Board Association in Washington, D.C.
11. Richard, *Has Sex Education Failed Our Teenagers?* 49.
12. Ibid., 18.
13. Jim Sedlak, research available from Stop Planned Parenthood, P.O. Box 8, LaGrangeville, NY 12540 (914-473-3316); Brad Hayton, *No Protection: The Failure of Condom-Based Sex Education,* Newport Beach, Calif.: Pacific Policy Institute, 1991 (714-723-6635); JacquelineKasun, "The Truth About Sex Education," in Barrett Mossbacher, *School-Based Clinics* (Westchester, Ill.: Crossway, 1987); "Teenage Pregnancy: What Comparisons Among States and Countries Show," (Stafford, Va.: American Life League, 1986); "The Baltimore School Birth Control Study: A Comment," Humbolt State University, 1; "The State and Adolescent Sexual Behavior," in Joseph R. Reden and Fred R. Glahe, eds., *The American Family and the State* (San Francisco: Pacific Research Institute for Public Policy, 1986).
14. *Psychology Today*, January/February 1989.
15. November 18, 1991, 11:00 P.M., PBS, Channel 18.
16. McDowell, *The Myths of Sex Education*, 16.
17. *Parents and Better Homemaking*, December 1965, 40.
18. McDowell, *The Myths of Sex Education*, 17.
19. Ibid., 22–23.

CHAPTER 2

1. "More Unsafe Sex," *U.S. News & World Report*, 1 October 1990; "Sex Habits of Young Women Change Little," *USA Today*, 16 March 1990 (citing a *New England Journal of Medicine* report).

2. Cochran and Mays, "Sex, Lies and HIV," *New England Journal of Medicine* 322, no. 11, 1991: 744 (correspondence); "Sex, Lies and Risk of AIDS,"*USA Today*, 15 March 1991, 1d (cf. *USA Today*, 15 August 1988 and 15 May 1986); Joe S. McIlhaney, *Sexuality and Sexually Transmitted Diseases* (Grand Rapids: Baker, 1990), 15; *USA Today*, 15 Aug. 1988, 1D.

3. Latest research from Dr. Robert Redfield, typed transcript of interview for "The John Ankerberg Show" (second interview), April 1992.

4. News Report on CNN, 18 December 1991.

5. C. S. Lewis, *Mere Christianity* (New York: Macmillan, 1971), 90–91.

6. Peggy Brick, et al. *Teaching Safer Sex* (Hackensack, N.J.: The Center for Family Life Education, Planned Parenthood of Bergen County, 1989), V.

7. Ibid.

8. Ibid., 27.

9. Ibid., 25.

10. Ibid., 26.

11. Ibid.

12. Ibid., 71.

13. Ibid., 34.

14. Ibid.

15. Ibid., 37–38.

16. Ibid., 41.

17. Ibid., X.

18. Ibid., V.

19. Ibid.,63–65.

20. Ibid., 75.

21. Ibid., 76.

22. See, e.g., The Planned Parenthood brochure (12 May 1989) announcing a family planning conference to be preceded by the safety dance developed by Jay Friedman, the same dance found in *Teaching Safer Sex*, 79–80. The program was sponsored by the Vermont Department of Health and Planned Parenthood of Northern New England.

23. Brick et al., *Teaching Safer Sex*, 80.

CHAPTER 3

1. Lorraine Day, *AIDS: What the Government Isn't Telling You* (Palm Desert, Calif.: Rockford, 1991), 233.

2. Asta Kenney, *Family Planning Perspectives*, January/February 1986, 6, 28; cited in Josh McDowell, *The Myths of Sex Education* (San Bernardino, Calif.: Here's Life, 1990), 61.

3. Wendell W. Hoffman and Stanley J. Grenz, *AIDS: Ministry in the Midst of An Epidemic* (Grand Rapids: Baker, 1990), 140.

4. Peter Gotzsche and Merete Hording et al., *Scandinavian Journal of Infectious Diseases* 20, from the Department of Infectious Diseases (Rigshospitalet, Copenhagen, Denmark, 1988), 202, 233–34, 252; cited in McDowell, *The Myths of Sex Education*, 62.

5. Day, *AIDS,* 232.

6. *Consumer Reports*, March 1989.

7. Hoffman and Grenz, AIDS, 139.

8. Ibid.

9. *New England Journal of Medicine*, 316, no. 21 (1987): 1339–42; cf. Margaret A. Fischl et al., "Evaluation of Heterosexual Partners, Children and Household Contacts of Adults with AIDS," *Journal of the American Medical Association*, 6 February 1987: 640–44; *Washington Post*, 6 February 1987.

10. Dinah Richard, *Has Sex Education Failed Our Teenagers? A Research Report* (Pomona, Calif.: Focus on the Family, 1990), 25.

11. Americans for a Sound AIDS/HIV Policy, *The Church's Reponse to the Challenge of AIDS/HIV: A Guideline for Education and Policy Development* (Washington, D.C., 1991), 31.

12. Kenney, *Family Planning Perspectives*, 6, 28.

13. Nicholas J. Fiumara, "Effectiveness of Condoms in Preventing VD," *New England Journal of Medicine*, 21 October 1971, 972.

14. Ibid.

15. Gotzsche et al., *Scandinavian Journal of Infectious Diseases*, 20: 223–24, 252.

16. S. E. Barton et al., "HTLV–123 Antibody in Prostitutes," *Lancet*, 21 December 1985, 1424.

17. *Dallas Times Herald*, 18 February 1989.

18. Interview with Dr. Robert Redfield conducted for "The John Ankerberg Show," typed transcript, 33.

19. Ibid.

20. *New York Times*, 18 August 1987.

21. Robert C. Noble "There Is No Safe Sex," *Newsweek*, 1 April 1991, 8.

22. "Condom Advertising," testimony before the House Subcommittee on Health and the Environment, 10 February 1987.

23. Edited transcript for "The John Ankerberg Show."

24. *New York Times*, 18 August 1987; telephone interview with staff of the Department of Education, Washington, D.C., 1 September 1987.

25. Thanks to Dr. Robert Redfield, interview conducted for "The John Ankerberg Show," typed transcript, 30–34.

26. J. J. Goedert, "What Is Safe Sex? Suggested Standards Linked to Testing for Human Immunodeficiency Virus," *New England Journal of Medicine*, 21 May 1987, 1339.

27. McDowell, *The Myths of Sex Education*, 65.

28. Sara Nelson, "Talking Smart, Acting Stupid About AIDS," *Glamour*, February 1992, 175.

29. Ibid., 191.

30. National Education Association, *The Facts About AIDS: A Special Guide for NEA Members* (1987), 16.

31. Robin Fox et al., "Changes In Sexual Activities Among Participants in the Multicenter AIDS Cohorts Study," Third International Conference on AIDS, Washington, D.C., Abstracts (June 1987), 213.

32. Ronald Valdiserri et al., "Condom Use in a Cohort of Gay and Bisexual Men," Third International Conference on AIDS.

33. Nelson, "Talking Smart," 174.

CHAPTER 4

1. Josh McDowell and Dick Day, *Why Wait? What You Need to Know About the Teen Sexuality Crisis* (San Bernardino, Calif.: Here's Life, 1987), 16.

2. Ibid., 17.

3. Dinah Richard, *Has Sex Education Failed Our Teenagers? A Research Report* (Pomona, Calif: Focus on the Family Publishing, 1990), 56–62.

4. Ibid. A list of nine abstinence-based curricula for public schools is found in Appendix C (cf. 54–57).

5. Josh McDowell, *Teens Speak Out: What I Wish My Parents Knew About My Sexuality* (San Bernardino, Calif.: Here's Life , 1991), 109–10.

6. *Parade*, 24 September 1989.

7. Josh McDowell, *The Myths of Sex Education* (San Bernardino, Calif.: Here's Life, 1990), 30.

8. Adapted from McDowell, *Teens Speak Out*, chap. 4.

CHAPTER 5

1. Joe S. McIlhaney, *Sexuality and Sexually Transmitted Diseases* (Grand Rapids: Baker, 1990), 10 (citing the American College of Obstetricians and Gynecologists). (Reprinted with the new title *Safe Sex: A Doctor Looks at the Risks and Realities of AIDS and Other STD's*).

2. Ibid., 15.

3. T. M. Hooten et al., "STD Briefs," *Medical Aspects of Human Sexuality*, February 1991, 59. This figure is also reported in the Boston Women's Health Book Collective, "STDs On the Rise," *Ms.*, March 1991, 76.

4. McIlhaney, *Sexuality*, 11; a partial listing of recent STD reports in popular magazines is illustrative, *Seventeen*, November 1990; *American Health*, May 1991, June 1991; *Glamour*, May 1991; *New York* magazine, 3 June 1991; *Scientific American*, March 1991; *Science*, 19 April 1991, 23 August 1991, 5 July 1991; *The Futurist*, March/April 1991; *World Health*, November/December 1990; *Discover*, February 1991; *Science News*, 20 April 1991.

5. William Hines, "Other Sex Diseases Dwarf AIDS," *Chicago Sun Times*, 21 May 1989, cites a figure of eighty thousand deaths from 1981.

6. Sevgi O. Aral and King K. Holmes, "Sexually Transmitted Diseases in the AIDS Era," *Scientific American*, February 1991, 62.

7. E.g., Jean Seligman, "A Nasty New Epidemic," *Newsweek*, 4 February 1985, 73.

8. Department of Continuing Education, Harvard Medical School, *The Harvard Medical School Health Letter*, April 1981, 1.

9. Judy Ismach, "Brave New World of Warts and Worries," *American Health*, April 1984, 84.

10. Ibid.

11. Ibid. This article noted that STDs were "the major cause of preventable sterility in American men and women" (p. 84). "In one decade, pelvic inflammatory disease from STDs has tripled the rate of ectopic pregnancies—to more than 50,000 a year. These tubal pregnancies require surgery to remove the embryo, and can kill the mother if not spotted early." The article further warned:

> STD-related complications—miscarriage, premature delivery, post-partum infection of the uterus, for instance—are only beginning to be documented. They probably affect over 100,000 women annually. At least 100,000 newborns a year have eye disease from chlamydial infection. Herpes from infected mothers kills hundreds of babies, though planned Caesarean birth will prevent it. Group B strep kills more babies each year than polio in any year before the vaccine. Those who live may be blind, deaf, retarded or have cerebral palsy. The list of STD/cancer ties is long and growing. Genital warts from papilloma viruses are strongly linked to cervical cancer and anal cancer in homosexual men, and hepatitis B is believed to be the leading cause of liver cancer (p. 86).

The article pointed out that germs and viruses can still get in men and women through infected condoms and that "all intra-uterine devices raise the risk of pelvic inflammatory disease, especially in the first four months use" (p. 87). The article noted that gonorrhea strains resistant to penicillin have "increased 13-fold in three years" (p. 88). Researchers are worried that they won't develop newer drugs quickly enough to keep ahead of resistant strains. Tests for many of these diseases such as chlamydia and ureaplasma are very costly and not always available.

12. Fifty-one of these diseases are mentioned in "Sharp Rise in Rare Sex Related Diseases," *New York Times*, Health Section, 14 July 1988; discovering a new one each nine months is mentioned in Lewis J. Lord, "Sex with Care," *U.S. News & World Report*, 2 June 1986; cf. McIlhaney, *Sexuality*, 97–167, who discusses twenty-two.

13. The Boston Women's Health Book Collective, *The New Ourbodies, Ourselves* (New York: Touchstone, 1984), 263.

14. Between the ages of twenty and thirty-five, according to Dr. Robert Francoeur, professor of Human Sexuality and Embryology in J. Kerby Anderson, *Genetic Engineering* (Grand Rapids: Zondervan, 1982), 23 (citing *Parents*, May 1981, 63–4).

15. *The New Ourbodies, Ourselves*, 265.

16. Statistics from the Center for Disease Control in Atlanta, from Josh McDowell, *The Myths of Sex Education* (San Bernardino, Calif.: Here's Life, 1990), 159; and Dinah Richard, *Has Sex Education Failed Our Teenagers? A Research Report* (Pomona, Calif.: Focus on the Family, 1990), 24; cf. *U.S. News & World Report*, 2 June 1986, 53; *American Health*, May 1991, 44; *Newsweek*, Summer/Fall, 1990, special issue, 57.

17. Ibid.; Peggy Brick et al., *Teaching Safer Sex* (Hackensack, N.J.: Center for Family Life Education, Planned Parenthood of Bergen County, Inc., 1989), 27.

18. Aral and Holmes, "Sexually Transmitted Diseases," 64.

19. Ibid., 66–67.

20. *Science News*, 6 April 1991, 215.

21. *Chicago Sun Times*, 21 May 1989.

22. *American Health*, May 1991, 44.

23. Ibid.

24. Richard, *Has Sex Education Failed Our Teenagers?* 24.

25. Cf. Curtis Pesman, "Love and Sex in the 90s: Our National Survey," *Seventeen*, November 1991.

26. *San Diego Union*, 7 October 1991, A1, A8 (citing CDC estimates, gives a figure of forty-three million).

27. McDowell, *The Myths of Sex Education*, 51.

28. *U.S. News & World Report*, 2 June 1986, 56.

29. Transcript of interview with Dr. Robert Redfield conducted on Jan. 30–31 and March 21, 1991.

30. CNN News report, 29 November 1991.

31. McDowell, *The Myths of Sex Education*, 160–61.

32. William H. Masters, Virginia E. Johnson, and Robert C. Kolodny, *Masters and Johnson on Sex and Human Loving* (Boston: Little, Brown, 1988), 535.

33. Ismach, "Brave New World," 46.

34. McIlhaney, *Sexuality*, 114 (citing *Journal of the American Medical Association*, 4 April 1986).

35. *Masters and Johnson on Sex and Human Loving*, 536.

36. McIlhaney, *Sexuality*, 114; *Masters and Johnson on Sex and Human Loving*, 537.

37. McDowell, *The Myths of Sex Education*, 51.

38. Aral and Holmes, "Sexually Transmitted Diseases," 66.

39. *Masters and Johnson on Sex and Human Loving*, 563.

40. Ibid., 564.

41. *The New OurBodies, Ourselves*, 264–65, 268–71.

42. "STD Briefs," *Medical Aspects of Human Sexuality*, December 1990, 53–54.

43. *Masters and Johnson on Sex and Human Loving*, 564.

44. Ismach, "Brave New World," 46.

45. Aral and Holmes, "Sexually Transmitted Diseases," 64.

46. *Masters and Johnson on Sex and Human Loving*, 566; *The New Ourbodies, Ourselves*, 265.

47. Ibid.

48. *Masters and Johnson on Sex and Human Loving*, 564.

49. Ibid.

50. McIlhaney, *Sexuality*, 24.

51. Wendy Gibbons, "Clueing in on Chlamydia: Microbial Stealth Leads to Reproductive Ravages," *Science News*, 20 April 1991, 250.

52. Ibid.

53. Aral and Holmes, "Sexually Transmitted Diseases," 66.

54. *Journal of the American Medical Association*, 23/30 January 1991, 475.

55. McIlhaney, *Sexuality*, 153–54.

56. Ibid.; cf. *Journal of the American Medical Association*, 23/30 January 1991, 475.

57. Ibid.; cf. Ting and Greer Bauer et al., "Nearly Half of Sexually Active College Women May Be HPV-Infected," *Medical Aspects of Human Sexuality*, March 1991, 49.

58. Ismach, "Brave New World," 46; cf. "STD's on the Rise," *Ms.*, 76.

59. See Aral and Holmes, "Sexually Transmitted Diseases," 66; *Journal of the American Medical Association*, 23/30 January 1991, 475; Ismach, "Brave New World," 46 (cf. "STD's on the Rise," *Ms.*, 76); McIlhaney, *Sexuality*, 136–39.

60. Ibid.

61. McIlhaney, *Sexuality*, 137.

62. Multiple sexual partners and beginning sexual intercourse at too early an age also increase a woman's chance for cervical cancer. Apparently, beginning sexual activity early is a greater risk than having multiple partners because of the immaturity of the cells that line the cervix in young women. "All studies agree that cervical cancer risk is increased by . . . first intercourse at early ages. By observing abstinence, the adolescent female is on reasonably valid biological grounds, which requires no moral or religious support" (*Journal of the American Medical Association*, 17 February 1962, 486; cited in McDowell, *Myths of Sex Education*, 170). One study discovered that the risk of cellular abnormalities of the cervix is five times greater in a group of promiscuous teenagers than among a group of virgin teenagers. The risk of cervical cancer doubles in women who become involved sexually before the age of seventeen (cf. McDowell, *Myths of Sex Education*, 170). Further, extramarital sexual practice by either the man or woman is also associated with cervical cancer risk.

63. "Epidemiology of Primary and Secondary Syphilis in the United States, 1981–1989," *Journal of the American Medical Association*, 19 September 1990, 1432; *U.S. News & World Report*, 14 August 1989, 7.

64. McIlhaney, *Sexuality*, 124–25, 128.

65. Ibid.

66. Ibid., 128–29.

67. *Journal of the American Medical Association*, 23/30 June 1989; *Washington Times*, 12 June 1989; *Washington Post*, 11 July 1989.

68. Ismach, "Brave New World," 46

69. Jonathan Zenilman, "Sexually Transmitted Diseases in Homosexual Adolescents," *Journal of Adolescent Health Care* 9, no. 2 (1988): 129–30.

70. McIlhaney, *Sexuality*, 165; cf. Joann M. Schulte et al., "Chancroid in the United States,

1981–1991: Evidence for Underreporting of Cases," Center for Disease Control, *Morbidity and Mortality Weekly Report* for 19 May 1992, pp. 57, 59.

71. *CMS Journal* 118 (Winter 1987): 28–30.

CHAPTER 6

1. Press release available from Harvard University, text to be published in late 1992; *International Healthwatch Report,* June 1992.

2. The following material is excerpted from Patrick Dixon, *The Whole Truth About AIDS* (Nashville: Nelson, 1989), 39–59, and Claudia Wallis, "Viruses," *Time*, 3 November 1986, 66–74.

3. Dixon, *The Whole Truth,* 54.

4. Ibid., 54; Lorraine Day "AIDS Risks," personal handout.

5. Dixon, *The Whole Truth,* 55–56.

6. Ibid., 57.

7. Ibid., 58–59.

8. Ibid., 40.

9. Ibid.; cf. *Scientific American* 255 (1986): 78–88, and 256 (1987): 38–48.

10. Dixon, *The Whole Truth,* 43.

11. *Time*, 3 November 1986; Wendell W. Hoffman and Stanley J. Gens, *AIDS: Ministry in the Midst of an Epidemic* (Grand Rapids: Baker, 1990), 64–67.

12. Dixon, *The Whole Truth,* 44.

13. Ibid.

14. Ibid., 45.

15. "The John Ankerberg Show," transcript of second interview, 19–21.

16. Dixon, *The Whole Truth,* 45.

17. Ibid.

18. *1989 World Almanac and Book of Facts* (New York: Pharos, 1988), 201.

19. Ibid., 52. For documentation see Gene Antonio, *AIDS: Rage and Reality: Why Silence is Deadly* (Dallas: Anchor, 1992), chaps 4–7.

20. William H. Masters, Virginia E. Johnson, and Robert C. Kolodny, *Masters and Johnson on Sex and Human Loving* (Boston: Little Brown, 1988), 549–50. See note 51.

21. "Dateline NBC," 14 April 1992, 10:00 P.M.

22. See note 1; Lorraine Day, *AIDS: What the Government Isn't Telling You* (Palm Desert, Calif.: Rockford, 1991), 210, 246; *U.S. News & World Report* (13 May 1991) cites thirty million adults and ten million children infected by the year 2000; according to the *Chattanooga News Free Press* (12 April 1992), the Asian Development Bank has forecast that Asia will account for most of the "projected fifty million cases" by 2000. (Other authorities have cited similar figures for Africa.) India and Thailand are especially vulnerable because of tolerance of prostitution.

23. Cf. Dixon, *The Whole Truth,* 19.

24. Day, *AIDS*, 169.

25. *USA Today*, 11 July 1990.

26. Day, *AIDS,* chap. 6.

27. Hoffman and Grenz, *AIDS: Ministry in the Midst of an Epidemic*, 84, 138; Day, *AIDS*, 158–62.

28. Day, AIDS, 161–62.

29. *1989 World Almanac*, 201.

30. John Weldon, "Homosexuality: Myths and Facts," *The Defender*, November 1989 (Chattanooga: Ankerberg Theological Research Institute), 1.

31. For several similar statements, see David A. Noebel et al., *AIDS: Special Report* (Manitow

Springs, Co.: Summit Research Institute, 1987), 34, 99, 174–78; e.g., Dr. Halfdon Mahler, director, World Health Organization, who said, "We stand nakedly in front of a very serious pandemic as mortal as any pandemic there ever has been. I don't know of any greater killer than AIDS" (*New York Times*, 21 November 1986); Dr. J. I. Slaff and J. K. Brubaker, who said, "The AIDS virus shows every sign of being just as deadly as the plague during the Middle Ages" (*The AIDS Epidemic*, 162); Dr. John Seale before California Senate Health and Human Services Committee (29 Sept. 1986), "The AIDS virus . . . has all that is needed to render the human race extinct within 50 years"; others have stated that without a cure or vaccine, up to half the world could be wiped out.

32. Dixon, *The Whole Truth*, 25.

33. Ibid., 37.

34. *1989 World Almanac*, 20.

35. *Dateline NBC*, 14 April 1991, 10:00 P.M., EST.

36. Day, *AIDS*, 150; cf. Paul Cameron, *Exposing the AIDS Scandal* (Lafayette, La.: Huntington, 1988), 45–63.

37. ISIS, "What Homosexuals Do," Institute for the Scientific Investigation of Sexuality, 1988 (2940 S. 74th St., Lincoln, NE 68506), 6.

38. ISIS, "Medical Aspects of Homosexuality," 5.

39. NBC News, 13 November 1991.

40. Day, *AIDS*, 164–65; cf. p. 159 and *New England Journal of Medicine*, 1 June 1989, 1458.

41. *JAMA Medical News*, 22/29 November 1985, 2866; Day, *AIDS*, 159.

42. Day, "AIDS Risks," handout, 1.

43. *Surgical Practice News*, August 1988, 15; "Surgical Glove Perforations," *British Journal of Surgery*, April 1988, 317.

44. *San Francisco Examiner*, 2 October 1987.

45. *San Francisco Chronical*, 15 June 1988, 4.

46. *Journal of the American Medical Association*, 16 December 1988, 3482; cf. *Science*, 16 June 1989.

47. *The Lancet*, 7 November 1987, 1094.

48. *Journal of the Royal Society of Medicine*, 78 (1975): 613–15.

49. *American Psychiatric Association Conference*, August 1989, New Orleans.

50. *The Lancet*, 20 September 1986, 694.

51. "Passionate Kissing and Microlesions of the Oral Mucosa: Possible Role in AIDS Transmission," *Journal of the American Medical Association*, 13 January 1989, 244–45; cf. *The Lancet*, 18 June 1988, 1395.

52. *Wall Street Journal*, 16 March 1986; Day, "AIDS Risks," 9. See Antonio, *AIDS*, chap. 7.

53. Day, "AIDS Risks," 3–6, 10.

54. Day, *AIDS*, 291.

55. Cf. Charles F. Turner et al., eds., *AIDS, Sexual Behavior and Intravenous Drug Use* (Washington, D.C.: National Academy, 1989), chap. 3.

56. Noted in the medical literature.

57. Personal conversations with Dr. Lorraine Day.

58. Cf. John Weldon, "Homosexuality," MS., 1992, passim.

59. See "The John Ankerberg Show," *Are There Other Ways HIV May Be Transmitted?* Program 4: "Eight Objections to Routine Testing."

60. Widely reported in the media, April 1992.

61. "AIDS Patient Guilty of Murder Try in Biting Policeman, Gets 10 Years," *Chattanooga News Free Press*, 22 October 1989.

62. Dixon, *The Whole Truth*, 110–11.

63. Ibid., 111.

64. Ibid.

65. Ibid., 108.

66. John Money, "Bisexual, Homosexual and Heterosexual: Society, Law and Medicine," *Journal of Homosexuality* (Spring 1977): 229.

67. Dixon, *The Whole Truth,* 112.

CHAPTER 7

1. Josh McDowell, *The Myths of Sex Education* (San Bernardino, Calif.: Here's Life, 1990), 48–49.

2. *Chicago Tribune,* 19 February 1986, 3.

3. Myron Harris and J. Norman, *The Private Life of the American Teenager* (New York: Rawson Wade , 1981), 99.

4. *USA Today,* 23 March 1989, 26; cited in McDowell, *The Myths of Sex Education,* 49.

5. Joe S. McIlhaney, *Sexuality and Sexually Transmitted Diseases* (Grand Rapids: Baker, 1990), 11 (citing *Journal of the American Medical Association,* 22/29 October 1982).

6. Nora Zamichow, *Times Herald;* cited in McDowell, *The Myths of Sex Education,* 50.

7. Some of these are from ibid., passim.

8. *The Common Appeal,* 7 November 1988, A12.

9. CNN News, 30 November 1991.

10. McDowell, *The Myths of Sex Education,* 53.

11. Ibid., 54; cf. Dinah Richard, *Has Sex Education Failed Our Teenagers? A Research Report* (Pomona, Calif.: Focus on the Family, 1990), 22, 28–29; Pearl Evans, *Hidden Danger in the Classroom* (Petaluma, Calif.: Small Helm, 1990),4–8.

12. McDowell, *The Myths of Sex Education,* 55 (citing AIDS Prevention, 1989, newsletter of the National AIDS Prevention Institute, Culpepper, Va.)

13. McDowell, *The Myths of Sex Education,* 55.

14. "Dateline NBC," 14 April 1992, 10:00 P.M., EST; *U.S. Newsweek Review,* 24 April 1989, 26.

15. Melvin Anchell, *What's Wrong with Sex Education?* (Selma, Al.: Hoffman Center for the Family, 1991), 85; cf. 74.

16. *Newsweek,* 1 December 1991. See "Multi-Drug Resistent Tuberculosis," Centers for Disease Control, *Morbidity and Mortality Weekly Report* for 19 June 1992.

17. *Journal of the American Family Association,* November/December 1991.

CHAPTER 8

1. William H. Masters, Virginia E. Johnson, Robert C. Kolodny, *Masters and Johnson on Sex and Human Loving* (Boston: Little, Brown, 1988), 10.

2. Pearl Evans, *Hidden Danger in the Classroom: Disclosure Based on Ideas of W. R. Coulson* (Petaluma, Calif.: Small Helm, 1990), 38–45.

3. Josh McDowell, *The Myths of Sex Education* (San Bernardino, Calif.: Here's Life, 1990), 40. An early 1992 editorial in the *Chattanooga News Free Press,* "Where TV Leads," cited 93 percent of network sex as pre- or extramarital.

4. Dinah Richard, *Has Sex Education Failed Our Teenagers? A Research Report* (Pomona, Calif.: Focus on the Family, 1990), 32.

5. "American Teens Speak: Sex, Myth, TV and Birth Control," The Planned Parenthood Poll, Lewis Harris and Associates, Inc., September/October 1986, 9; cited in McDowell, *The Myths of Sex Education,* 41.

6. Elizabeth F. Brown and William Hendee, "Adolescents and Their Music: Insights into the Health of Adolescents," *Journal of the American Medical Association,* 22/29 September 1989, 1659.

7. E.g., Liebert, Sprafkin, and Davidson, *The Early Window: Effects of Television on Children and Youth* (1982), 171; cited in Josh McDowell and Dick Day, *Why Wait? What You Need to Know About the Teen Sexuality Crisis* (San Bernardino, Calif.: Here's Life, 1987), 40.

8. McDowell, *The Myths of Sex Education*, 39.

9. Ibid.

10. Virginia Anderson and Randolph Allen Wright, "The Impact of Media on the Sexual Attitudes of Adolescents," a paper presented at the New Orleans, La., Conference, 5-8 November 1989; cited in McDowell, *The Myths of Sex Education*, 39.

11. McDowell, *The Myths of Sex Education*, 38.

12. Ibid.

13. Anderson and Wright, "The Impact of the Media," 6.

14. McDowell and Day, *Why Wait?* 40.

15. McDowell, *The Myths of Sex Education*, 47.

CHAPTER 9

1. Brad Hayton, *No Protection: The Failure of Condom-Based Sex Education* (Newport Beach, Calif.: Pacific Policy Institute, 1991), 2.

2. Dinah Richard, *Has Sex Education Failed Our Teenagers? A Research Report* (Pomona, Calif.: Focus on the Family, 1990), III.

3. Joseph A. Olsen and Stan Weed, "Effects of Family-Planning Programs for Teenagers on Adolescent Birth and Pregnancy Rates," and "Effects of Family-Planning Programs on Teenage Pregnancy-Replication and Extension," *Family Perspectives* (Fall 1986): 154–95; cf. *Wall Street Journal*, 14 October 1986; cited in Richard, *Has Sex Education Failed Our Teenagers?* 6.

4. Richard, *Has Sex Education Failed Our Teenagers?* 8.

5. Ibid., 11.

6. Cited in ibid., 19.

7. Review of Peter R. Kilman et al., "Sex Education: A Review of Its Effects," *Archives of Sexual Behavior* 10, no. 2 (1981): 177–205, in *Family Life Educator*, Preview issue, May 1982: 27; cited in Richard, *Has Sex Education Failed Our Teenagers?* 22.

8. Richard, *Has Sex Education Failed Our Teenagers?* 20–22.

9. A. Pietropinto, "A Survey on Contraception Analysis," *Medical Aspects of Human Sexuality*, May 1987: 147; cited in Richard, *Has Sex Education Failed Our Teenagers?* 11.

10. Melvin Zelnik and Young J. Kim, "Sex Education and Its Association with Teenage Sexual Activity, Pregnancy, and Contraceptive Use," *Family Planning Perspectives*, May/June 1982: 117–26; cited in Richard, *Has Sex Education Failed Our Teenagers?* 19.

11. Richard, *Has Sex Education Failed Our Teenagers?* 22.

12. Melvin Anchell, "Psychoanalysis vs. Sex Education," *National Review*, 20 June 1986, 33.

13. Quoted in Sean O'Reilly, *Sex Education in the Schools* (Thaxton, Va: Sun Life, 1978); cited in Richard, *Has Sex Education Failed Our Teenagers?* 28.

14. Ibid.

15. Richard, *Has Sex Education Failed Our Teenagers?* 29 (citing Joseph R. Peden and Fred R. Glahe,, eds., *The American Family* [San Francisco: Pacific Research Institute for Public Policy, 1986], 357).

16. Wanda Franz, "Adolescent Cognitive Abilities and Implications for Sexual Decision Making," paper presented at Celebrate the Family, Third Eastern Symposium, Pennsylvania State Univ., 24 March 1987; cited in Richard, *Has Sex Education Failed Our Teenagers?* 31.

17. Anchell, "Psychoanalysis vs. Sex Education," 33, 38.

18. Ibid.

19. Ibid.

20. Ibid.

21. Ibid.

22. Wardell B. Pomeroy, *Girls and Sex* (New York: Delacorte-Dell, 1991), 100.

23. Wardell B. Pomeroy, *Boys and Sex* (New York: Delacorte-Dell, 1991), 99–100.

24. Richard, *Has Sex Education Failed Our Teenagers?* 27; cf. the research of associate professor of sociology Nancy Moore Clatworth (Ohio State Univ.) reported in "Prior Cohabitation Linked to Unsuccessful Marriages," *Los Angeles Times*, 21 November 1976.

25. Anchell, "Psychoanalysis vs. Sex Education," 60.

26. Douglas Kirby, speaking at the 16th annual meeting of the National Planning and Reproductive Health Association, 2 March 1988, Washington, D.C., session, education, audio tape recording and transcript by Richard Glasow; the final report promised by Kirby had not yet been published; cited in McDowell, *The Myths of Sex Education* (San Bernardino, Calif.: Here's Life, 1990), 112, 290.

27. McDowell, *The Myths of Sex Education*, chap. 9.

28. Ibid.

29. Ibid., 120.

30. Ibid., 121; cf. chap. 10.

31. Debra A. N. Dawson, "The Effects of Sex Education on Adolescent Intercourse, Contraception and Pregnancy in the United States," *Family Planning Perspectives*, July/August 1986: 168–69.

32. McDowell, *The Myths of Sex Education*, 135.

33. Ibid., 138.

34. Anne Newman and Dinah Richard, *Health Sex Education in Your Schools* (Colorado Springs: Focus on the Family, 1990).

CHAPTER 10

1. Josh McDowell, *The Myths of Sex Education* (San Bernardino, Calif.: Here's Life, 1990), 82.

2. Ibid., 83, cf. William Bennett, "Sex and the Education of Our Children," in Barrett Mosbacker, "Teen Pregnancy in School-Based Health Clinics," *Vision*, October/November, 1986: 162.

3. A. M. Morgan, "Comprehensive Sex-Ed: Ten Fatal Flaws," Virginians for Family Values, n.d.

4. W. R. Coulson, "Founder of Value-Free Education Says He Owes Parents an Apology," *American Family Association Journal*, April 1989: 21–22.

5. Alexandra and Vernon Mark, *The Pied Pipers of Sex* (Plainfield, N.J.: Haven Books, 1981), 26.

6. McDowell, *The Myths of Sex Education*, 87.

7. Wardell B. Pomeroy, *Boys and Sex* (New York: Delacorte-Dell, 1991), 1–2.

8. Ibid., 13.

9. Wardell B. Pomeroy, *Girls and Sex* (New York: Delacorte-Dell, 1991), 5.

10. Pomeroy, *Boys*, 105.

11. Pomeroy, *Girls*, 1; cf. *The Hite Reports* on male and female sexuality.

12. Pomeroy, *Girls*, 2.

13. Ibid., 3.

14. Ibid., 12.

15. Ibid., 16.

16. Ibid., 68–69.

17. Ibid., 92–3.

18. Ibid., 53.
19. Ibid., 100–101.
20. Ibid., 101.
21. Ibid., 157–58.
22. Pomeroy, *Boys*, 4.
23. Ibid., 13.
24. Ibid., 9.
25. Ibid., 5–6.
26. Ibid., 10–11.
27. Ibid., 17.
28. Ibid., 2.
29. Ibid., 83.
30. Ibid., 177.
31. Ibid., 144–45.
32. Ibid., 145.
33. Ibid., 165.
34. Ibid., 99–100.
35. Ibid., 101.
36. Ibid., 84.
37. Ibid., 51–52, 60.
38. Ibid., 106–12.
39. Marilyn Ratner and Susan Shamlin, *Straight Talk: Sexuality Education for Parents and Kids,* 4–7 (New York: Penguin Books for Planned Parenthood, 1988).
40. Pomeroy, *Boys*, 56–57.
41. Ibid., 161.
42. Ibid., 62.
43. McDowell, *The Myths of Sex Education,* 88.
44. Ibid., 97; confirmed by our research in New York, April 1992.
45. McDowell, *The Myths of Sex Education,* 96.
46. Ibid., p. 97.
47. Ibid., 98–100.
48. "Teens and AIDS," published by the division of AIDS Program Services, New York, City Department of Health and funded by the Centers for Disease Control and the City of New York, January 1991.
49. McDowell, *The Myths of Sex Education,* 100.

CHAPTER 11

1. Josh McDowell, *Teens Speak Out: What I Wish My Parents Knew About My Sexuality* (San Bernardino, Calif.: Here's Life, 1991), 84.
2. *The Conservative Book Club,* List No. 1391.
3. Dinah Richard, *Has Sex Education Failed Our Teenagers? A Research Report* (Pomona, Calif.: Focus on the Family, 1990), 26.
4. "Saturday Night with Connie Chung," 18 November 1989; initial transcript, 5.
5. "Exclusive Interview: U.S. Surgeon General C. Everett Koop," *Rutherford Journal* (Manassas, Va.: The Rutherford Institute, Spring 1989), 30–7; Robert G. Marshall, *Dissolving Compromise by the Study of Truth* (Stafford, Va.: American Lifeleague, Inc., n.d.); cf. "Dr. Koop's Non Report," 5, end pages.

6. Vincent M. Rue et al., *A Report on the Psychological Aftermath of Abortion* (presented to C. Everett Koop by the National Right to Life Committee), 15 September 1987, Washington, D.C., 5. Appendix One summarizes ninety studies.

7. Thomas W. Hilgers and Dennis J. Horan, *Abortion and Social Justice* (Thaxton, Va: Sun Life, 1980), 58, 77.

8. See American Rights Coalition (pamphlet), *The Abortion Injury Report,* September 1989, 2 (1-800-634-2224); Wanda Franz, Testimony, U.S. Congress, House, Human Resources and Intergovernmental Relations Subcommittee of the Committee on Government Operations, hearing on *Medical and Psychological Impact of Abortion,* 101 Cong., First Session, 16 March 1989. See also Vincent Rue, *The Hatch Hearings,* vol. 1, 329–78; N. Spreckhard, *The Psycho-Social Stress Following Abortion* (Kansas City, Mo.: Sheed & Ward, 1987); N. Spreckhard, ed., *Post-Abortion Trauma* (1987); David Mall and Walter F. Watts, M.D., eds., *Psychological Aspects of Abortion* (Frederick, Md.: University Publications of America, 1979); David Reardon, *Aborted Women: Silent No More* (Westchester, Ill.: Crossway, 1987), 89–114; The Rutherford Institute, *Major Articles and Books Concerning the Detrimental Effects of Abortion* (summary report from hundreds of scientific studies published in medical and psychological journals), Manassas, Va.: The Rutherford Institute, 1990; additional sources are cited in Ankerberg and Weldon, *When Does Life Begin? And 39 Other Tough Questions About Abortion* (Dallas: Word, 1990), 2, 33.

9. Debra Evans, Without Moral Limits: Women, Reproduction and the New Medical Technology (Westchester, Ill.: Crossway, 1989), 60–61.

10. See note 8.

11. National Right to Life Educational Trust Fund, "Abortion: Some Medical Facts" (Washington, D.C., NRLETF, 1989), 5 (pamphlet).

12. Reardon, *Aborted Women*, 93.

13. Ibid., 96.

14. Ibid., 97.

15. Ibid., 99.

16. Ibid., 100–101.

17. Ibid., 106–077.

18. Ibid., 109–11.

19. Ibid., 108–13.

20. Carol Everett, "What I Saw in the Abortion Industry" (Jefferson City, Mo.: Easton, 1988) (pamphlet); Reardon, *Aborted Women*, 232–72.

21. Reardon, *Aborted Women,* 142.

22. Anne Catherine and Speckhard, "Psycho/Social Aspects of Stress Following Abortion," (Ph.D. diss., Univ. of Minnesota, 1985; cited in McDowell, *Teens Speak Out,* 178–79).

23. Reardon, *Aborted Women*, 119.

24. "Exclusive Interview: U.S. Surgeon General C. Everett Koop," 32–33.

25. Ibid., 31.

26. Marshall, *Dissolving Compromise,* passim.

27. "Exclusive Interview: U.S. Surgeon General C. Everett Koop," *Rutherford Journal* (Spring 1989), 33.

28. Paul Fowler, *Abortion: Toward An Evangelical Consensus* (Portland, Oreg.: Multnomah, 1987), 196.

29. Interview with Coleman McCarthy, "Does Abortion Harden Maternal Instinct?" National Catholic Reporter, 24 February 1989, 20.

30. Reardon, *Aborted Women,* 116.

31. Vincent M. Rue, et al., *A Report on the Psychological Aftermath of Abortion,* 53; cf., *Chattanooga News Free Press,* 4 Sept. 1992, 1.

32. E.g., ibid., 8–11.

33. Reardon, *Aborted Women*, 115.

34. Ibid., 116–17.

35. Ibid., 119–20.

36. Ibid., 129.

37. Ibid., 130–31.

38. Ibid., 134–35.

39. Vincent M. Rue et al., *Psychological Aftermath*, passim; Wanda Franz, Testimony; see note 8.

40. Vincent M. Rue et al., *Psychological Aftermath*, 4.

41. National Right to Life Educational Trust Fund, "Abortion: Some Medical Facts," 7.

42. Ibid., 5.

43. Vincent M. Rue et al., *Psychological Aftermath*.

44. Ibid., 11. Discovery, verification, and large scale epidemiological assessment are usually the three phases of research progression. This report noted that in the case of the postabortion reactions only the first phase of research had been conducted, with the observation that the need for phase two has been demonstrated and the recommendation that it proceed. 45. Ibid., 53.

46. Ibid., 8.

47. Ibid., 7.

48. Ibid., 6–7.

49. Ibid., 53.

50. Ibid., 54.

51. Ibid., Appendix 1.

CHAPTER 12

1. Judith A. Reisman et al., *Kinsey, Sex and Fraud: The Indoctrination of a People* (Lafayette, La.: Huntington, 1990), 4.

2. Ibid., 1.

3. Ibid., 2, first italics added.

4. E.g., Reisman et al., *Kinsey, Sex and Fraud*, 14; Thomas Weyr, *Reaching for Paradise: The Playboy Vision of America* (New York: Time Books, 1987), 11.

5. Reisman et al., *Kinsey, Sex and Fraud*, 1.

6. Ibid., 2.

7. Ibid., 117.

8. Ibid., 20–21.

9. John Court, in Reisman et al., *Kinsey, Sex and Fraud*, viii.

10. Reisman et al., *Kinsey, Sex and Fraud*, 3.

11. Ibid., 216.

12. Ibid., 7.

13. Ibid.

14. Ibid., 8.

15. Ibid., 17.

16. Ibid., 3, 6.

17. Ibid., 3.

18. Ibid.

19. Ibid., 15.

20. Ibid.

21. Ibid., 13; cf. Patrick J. Buchanan, "Sex Revolution Has Flimsy Basis," *Houston Chronicle*, 20 Oct. 1990, who cites the 31st annual conference of the Society for the Scientific Study of Sex where a sex expert argued that pedophiles also have "sexual rights."

22. Ibid., 4.

23. Ibid., 11; cf. Appendix D.

24. According to research from the Family Research Institute, Washington, D.C.

25. Reisman et al., *Kinsey, Sex and Fraud*, 225 citing *Time*, 14 April 1980.

26. Ibid.

27. Reisman et al., *Kinsey, Sex and Fraud*, 3.

28. Ibid.,3–4; cf. chap. 4.

29. In March 1992, cf. Robert Marshall and Charles Donovan, *Blessed Are the Barren: The Social Policy of Planned Parenthood* (San Francisco: Ignatius, 1991), 66–78.

30. Reisman et al., *Kinsey, Sex and Fraud*, 220.

31. Dinah Richard, *Has Sex Education Failed Our Teenagers? A Research Report* (Pomona, Calif.: Focus on the Family, 1990), 18.

32. Ibid., 11.

33. Marshall and Donovan, *Blessed Are the Barren*, 96.

34. Ibid., 320.

35. Ibid., back cover.

36. Ibid., ix.

37. Ibid., 1, 8–10, 60–63.

38. Ibid., 5–7.

39. Ibid., 7.

40. Ibid., 131.

41. Ibid., 321.

CHAPTER 13

1. Amici Curiae brief in Bowers v. Hardwick, 1986; cited in Family Research Institute, "Medical Consequences of What Homosexuals Do" (Washington, D.C.: Family Research Institute, 1992), 1.

2. Paul Cameron, *Family Research Report*, March/April, 1992, passim.

3. Paul Cameron, *Family Research Report*, April/June 1991, 7.

4. Family Research Institute, "Medical Consequences of What Homosexuals Do," 4–5.

5. John F. Harvey, *The Homosexual Person: New Thinking in Pastoral Care* (San Francisco: Ignatius, 1987), 103 (citing *Commentary*, January 1979, 20–22; cf. Ronald Lawler, Joseph Boyle, Jr., William E. May, *Catholic Sexual Ethics*, Huntington, Ind.: Our Sunday Visitor, 1985), 269.

6. ISIS, "The Psychology of Homosexuality," Institute for the Scientific Investigation of Sexuality, 1988 (2940 S. 74th St., Lincoln, Neb.. 85406), 6.

7. John Rechy, *The Sexual Outlaw: A Documentary* (New York: Grove, 1972), 300.

8. *1989 World Almanac and Book of Facts* (New York: Pharos/St. Martin's, 1988), 201.

9. "Increased Risk of Suicide in Persons with AIDS," *Journal of the American Medical Association* 259, no. 9 (1988).

10. Patrick Dixon, *The Whole Truth About AIDS* (Nashville, Tenn.: Thomas Nelson, 1989), 109.

11. Ibid., 105.

12. Ibid.

13. The Family Research Institute, *Family Research*, (Summer 1989): 1–6.

14. Manuscript of taped interview for "The John Ankerberg Show."

15. ISIS, "The Psychology of Homosexuality," 2.

16. John Jefferson Davis, *Evangelical Ethics: Issues Facing the Church Today* (Phillipsburg, N.J.: Presb. & Ref., 1985), 113.

17. ISIS, "Medical Aspects of Homosexuality," 1988, 2–3.

18. Family Research Institute, "Medical Consequences of What Homosexuals Do," 4 (pamphlet).

19. Paul Cameron et al., "Sexual Orientation and Sexually Transmitted Diseases," *The Nebraska Medical Journal*, August 1985, 292.

20. Ibid., 297–98.

21. J. R. Daling, "Sexual Practices, STD's and the Incidents of Anal Cancer," *New England Journal of Medicine* 317 (1987): 973.

22. William F. Owen, Jr., "Sexually Transmitted Diseases and Traumatic Problems in Homosexual Men," *Annals of Internal Medicine* 92 (1980): 805.

23. Ibid.

24. Ibid.

25. Ibid., 806.

26. Ibid.

27. Ibid.

28. Ibid., 805, 807.

29. Paul Cameron, *Exposing the AIDS Scandal* (LaFayette, La.: Huntington, 1988), 39.

30. ISIS, "Child Molestation and Homosexuality," 1988, 3.

31. Ibid., 1.

32. Ibid., 3.

33. Ibid., 6. The original research for this is found in Paul Cameron, "Homosexual Molestation of Children/Sexual Interaction of Teacher and Pupil," *Psychological Reports* 57 (1985); and in Paul Cameron et al., "Child Molestation and Homosexuality," *Psychological Reports* 58 (1986).

34. Cf. *The Washington Times*, 27 May 1992; cited in *Family Research Report*, January/February 1992: 5.

35. Lorraine Day, *AIDS: What the Government Isn't Telling You* (Palm Desert, Calif.: Rockford, 1991), 66.

36. The Family Research Institute, *Family Research* (Summer 1989): 5.

37. Paul Cameron, *Exposing the AIDS Scandal*, 122–23; Day, *AIDS,* passim.

38. ISIS, "Medical Aspects of Homosexuality," 7.

39. E.g., Day, *AIDS,* 65.

40. E.g., see the illustration in Paul Cameron, "A Case vs. Homosexuality," *The Human Life Review* (Summer 1978): 40.

41. William Dannemeyer, *Shadow in the Land: Homosexuality in America* (San Francisco: Ignatius, 1989), 102.

42. Cited *Family Research Report*, January/February 1992, 1, 5.

43. In ISIS, "What Homosexuals Do," 1988, 5; cited in *Executive Intelligence Report*, 18 October 1985.

44. Paul Cameron and Kirk Cameron, "Did the American Psychological Association Misrepresent Scientific Material to the U.S. Supreme Court?" *Psychological Reports* 63 (1988):1.

45. Cf. Dominick Vetri, "The Legal Arena: Progress for Gay Civil Rights," *Journal of Homosexuality* (Fall/Winter 1979–80): 25–32.

46. ISIS, "Criminality, Social Disruption and Homosexuality," 1988, 2.

47. Ibid.

48. Ibid., 3–5.
49. ISIS, "Murder, Violence and Homosexuality," 1988, 2.
50. Ibid., 4–5.
51. Cited in *Family Research Report*, January/February 1992, 1 (citing *The Wanderer*, 16 November 1991).
52. ISIS, "Murder, Violence and Homosexuality," 6.
53. Paul Cameron, Kirk Cameron, and Kay Proctor, "Homosexuality in the Armed Forces," *Psychological Reports* 62 (1988): 211.
54. Kirk Cameron and Kay Proctor, "Effect of Homosexuality upon Public Health and Social Order," *Psychological Reports* 64 (1989): 1167.
55. Ibid., 1177; cf. Table One, 1171–74.
56. ISIS, "Criminality, Social Disruption and Homosexuality," 6 (citing W. L. Shirer, *The Nightmare Years: 1939–1940* [1984] and L. Weddington, "The Role of Gay Activists in the Rise of Nazi Germany," *New York Tribune*, 1 September 1984).
57. John Stott, "Homosexual Partnerships," in *Involvement: Social and Sexual Relationships in the Modern World*, vol. 2 (Old Tappan, N.J.: Revell, 1985), 13.
58. Roger Montgomery, *My Life in Homosexuality* (MS, 1989), 25–7.
59. Gerhard van den Aardweg, *Homosexuality and Hope: A Psychologist Talks About Treatment and Change* (Ann Arbor, Mich.: Servant, 1988), 8–9.
60. Ibid., 20–21.
61. Ibid., 19.
62. Ibid., 18.
63. Paul Cameron and Kenneth P. Ross, "Social Psychological Aspects of the Judeo-Christian Stance Towards Homosexuality," *Journal of Psychology and Theology* (Spring 1981): 56.
64. Aardweg, *Homosexuality and Hope*, 22.
65. Oprah Winfrey transcript, no. 803 (11 October 1989), 9.
66. Ibid., 3.
67. John Weldon, "Homosexuality, " MS, 1991.

APPENDIX 2

1. Kim Painter, "Religions: AIDS Isn't God's Wrath," *USA Today*, 2 October 1989 (citing J. Gordon Melton, *The Churches Speak on AIDS* [New York: Gale Research, 1989]).
2. Margaret Clarkson, *Destined for Glory: The Meaning of Sufffering* (Grand Rapids: Eerdmans, 1983), 75.
3. Wendell W. Hoffman and Stanley J. Grenz, *AIDS: Ministry in the Midst of an Epidemic* (Grand Rapids: Baker, 1990), 165.
4. Ibid., 169.
5. Ibid., 170.
6. Ibid.
7. Ibid., 166.

Select Bibliography

Books

Adolescent Sexuality: Special Subject Bibliography January–December 1991. New York: Planned Parenthood Federation of America, Inc., 1992.

Anchell, Melvin, M.D. *What's Wrong With Sex Education?* Selma, Al.: Hoffman Center for The Family, 1991.

Blank, Joani and Marcia Quackenbush. *A Kid's First Book About Sex.* Burlingame, Calif.: Yes Press, 1983.

The Boston Women's Health Book Collective. *The New Our Bodies, Ourselves: A Book by and for Women.* New York: Simon & Schuster, 1984.

Brick, Peggy, and Carolyn Cooperman. *Positive Images: A New Approach to Contraceptive Education.* 2d. ed. Hackensack, NJ: The Center for Family Life Education, Planned Parenthood of Bergen County, Inc., 1987.

Bell, Ruth et al. *Changing Bodies Changing Lives.* New York: Vintage, 1987.

Brick, Peggy, with Catherine Charlton, Hillary Kunins, and Steve Brown. *Teaching Safer Sex.* Hackensack, N.J.: Center for Family Life Education, 1989.

Bundy, Patty, M.Ed., Susan McDonald, Ed.D., Janet McDowell, Ph.D. *Partners in Diversity: Planned Parenthood at Work With Religious Congregations.* Roanoke: Planned Parenthood of Southwest Virginia, Inc., 1988.

Callen, Michael, ed. *Surviving and Thriving With AIDS: Collected Wisdom, Vol. Two.* New York: People with AIDS Coalition, Inc., 1988.

Cameron, Paul, Ph.D. *Exposing the AIDS Scandal.* Lafayette, La.: Huntington House, Inc., 1988.

Cases of AIDS in Your Neighborhood—Queens—Cumulative Adult AIDS Cases By Race, Gender, Age and Risk Factor in New York City—August 1990. New York: AIDS Program Services, New York City Department of Health, 1990.

Child Abuse in the Classroom. Excerpts from official transcript of proceedings before the U.S. Department of Education. Edited by Phyllis Schlafly. Westchester, Ill.: Crossway, 1985.

Choices. . . . Denver: RAJ Publications/1982 by Pointed Publications, 1982.

The Church's Response to the Challenge of AIDS/HIV: A Guideline - for Education and Policy Development. Washington, D.C.: Americans for a Sound AIDS/HIV Policy, 1991.

Evans, Pearl. *Hidden Danger in the Classroom.* Petaluma, Calif.: Small Helm Press, 1990.

First Facts: A Manual for Sexuality Educators. New York: Education Department, Planned Parenthood Federation of America, Inc., 1986.

Geisler, Norman L. *Christian Ethics.* Grand Rapids: Baker, 1989.

Gitchel Sam and Lorri Foster. *Let's Talk About . . . s-e-x.* Fresno, Calif.: Planned

Parenthood of Central California, 1989.

A 'Guidebook' for National Family Sexuality Education Month. New York: Education Department/Planned Parenthood Federation of America, Inc., 1981.

A 'Guidebook' Supplement for National Family Sexuality Education Month. New York: Education Department/Planned Parenthood Federation of America, Inc., 1986.

Hayton, Brad. *No Protection: The Failure of Condom-Based Sex Education.* Pacific Policy Institute, 1991.

Highlights of the PPFA Issues Manual: A Guide for Planned Parenthood Volunteers. New York: Resource Division, Planned Parenthood Federation of America, Inc., nd.

Hite, Shere. *The Hite Report on Male Sexuality.* New York: Ballantine, 1981.

Hoffman, Wendell W., and Stanley J. Grenz. *AIDS: Ministry in the Midst of an Epidemic.* Grand Rapids: Baker, 1990.

– – –. *The Hite Report: A Nationwide Study of Female Sexuality.* New York: Dell, 1981.

Koch, Mayor Edward I., and Stephen C. Joseph, M.D., M.P.H., Commissioner. *AIDS: A Resource Guide for New York City.* New York: Department of Public Health, 1989.

The Lesbian & Gay Community Services Center. New York: LGCSC, Inc., 1990.

Madaras, Lynda. *The What's Happening to My Body? Book for Boys.* New York: Newmarket, 1988.

– – –. *The What's Happening to My Body? Book for Girls.* New York: Newmarket, 1988.

Marshall, Robert, Charles Donovan. *Blessed Are the Barren.* San Francisco: Ignatius, 1991.

Masters, William H., Virginia E. Johnson, and Robert C. Kolodny. *Masters and Johnson on Sex and Human Loving.* Boston: Little, Brown, 1985.

McDowell, Josh. *The Myths of Sex Education.* San Bernardino: Here's Life, 1990.

– – –. *Research Almanac & Statistical Digest.* Josh D. McDowell, 1991.

– – –. *Teens Speak Out: "What I Wish My Parents Knew About My Sexuality".* San Bernardino: Here's Life, 1987.

– – –. *Why Wait?.* San Bernardino: Here's Life, 1987.

McIlhaney, Joe S., Jr., M.D. *Safe Sex.* Grand Rapids: Baker, 1990. Reprinted as *Sexuality and Sexually Transmitted Diseases.* Grand Rapids: Baker, 1991.

Newman, Anne, and Dinah Richard. *Healthy Sex Education in Your Schools.* Colorado Springs: Focus on the Family, 1990.

Noebel, David A., Wayne C. Lutton, and Paul Cameron. *AIDS: Acquired Immune Deficiency Syndrome Special Report.* Manitou Springs, Co.: Summit Research Institute, 1986.

Ortiz, Elizabeth Thompson, *Your Complete Guide to Sexual Health.* Englewood Cliffs, N.J.: Prentice-Hall, 1989.

Pence, David M., M.D.,and Philip B. Sackett, Ph.D. *Values in Public Education.* St. Paul, Minn. Berean League, 1989.

Pomeroy, Wardell B., Ph.D. *Boys and Sex.* 3d ed. New York: Delacorte/Dell, 1991.

– – –. *Girls and Sex.* 3d ed. New York: Delacorte/Dell, 1991.

Programs in Place: Planned Parenthood Affiliate Programs for Adolescents. New York: Planned Parenthood Federation of America, Inc., 1990.

Ratner, Marilyn, and Susan Chamlin. *Straight Talk: Sexuality Education for Parents and Kids 4-7.* New York: Penguin Books for Planned Parenthood, 1988.

Redman, Julie M. *Women and AIDS: What We Need to Know.* New Orleans: Planned Parenthood of Louisiana, 1990.

Reisman, Dr. Judith A., and Edward W. Eichel. *Kinsey, Sex and Fraud: The Indoctrination of a People.* Edited by Drs. John H. Court & J. Gordon Muir. Lafayette, La.: Lochinvar/Huntington House Publishers, 1990.

Roberts, Gloria A. *A Family Planning Library Manual*. New York: Planned Parenthood Federation of America, Inc., 1982.

Sanchez, Ellen, M.Ed. *Which of These Teens Has AIDS?* Austin: Planned Parenthood of Austin, Inc., n.d.

Scott, Douglas R. *Inside Planned Parenthood*. Falls Church, Va.: CAC, 1990.

75 Years of Family Planning in America: A Chronology of Major Events. New York: Planned Parenthood Federation of America, 1991.

Tepper, Sheri B. *So You Don't Want To Be a Sex Object*. N.p., n.d. photocopy.

A Tradition of Choice for 75 Years—1991 Service Report. New York: Planned Parenthood Federation of America, Inc., 1991.

Young, Curt. *The Least of These*. Chicago: Moody, 1984.

Pamphlets, Periodicals and Miscellaneous

AIDS and Adolescents: A Resource Listing for Parents and Professionals. Reference Sheet #11. New York: Education Department Planned Parenthood of America, Inc., n.d.

Barton, S. E. et al. "HTLV-123 Antibody in Prostitutes." *Lancet*, 21 December 1985, 1424. (Up to 50 percent failure rate of condoms in male homosexual activity.)

The Boston Women's Health Book Collective. "STDs on the Rise." *Ms*. March–April 1991.

Cox, Harvey. "Brave New World of Warts and Worries." *American Health*, April 1984.

Department of Continuing Education, Harvard Medical School. "Sexually Transmitted Diseases." *The Harvard Medical School Health Letter*, April 1981.

Facklemann, K. A. "Virus—Smoking Synergy Causes Malignancy." *Science News*, 6 April 1991.

Fischl, M. A., et al. "Evaluation of Heterosexual Partners, Children, and Household Contacts of Adults With AIDS." *Journal of the American Medical Association*, 6 February 1987.

Friend, Tim. "Women's Death Rate From AIDS Is Soaring." *USA Today*, 11 July 1990.

"Genital Herpes and Acyclovir." *The Medical Forum, Harvard Medical School Health Letter*. September 1982.

Gibbons, Wendy. "Clueing in on Clamydia: Microbial Stealth Leads to Reproductive Ravages." *Science News*, 20 April 1991.

Health Section. "Sharp Rise in Rare Sex Related Diseases." *The New York Times*, 14 July 1988.

Hersch, Patricia. "Sexually Transmitted Diseases Are Ravaging Our Children, Teen Epidemic." *American Health*, May 1991.

Hooten, T. M., S. Hillier, C. Johnson et al. "STD Briefs." *Medical Aspects of Human Sexuality*, February 1991.

Jolata, Gina. "AIDS Researchers Settle in for Long Haul." *International Herald Tribune*, 6 June 1991.

"More Girls Having Sex as Teens." *USA Today*. November 8, 1990.

"More Unsafe Sex." *U.S. News & World Report*, 1 October 1990.

Nelson, Sara. "Talking Smart, Acting Stupid About AIDS." *Glamour*, February 1992.

New Woman, October 1987.

Newcomber, Susan, Ph.D. *Does Sexuality Education Make a Difference?* New York: Department of Education Planned Parenthood Federation of America, Inc., n.d.

Noble, Robert C. "The Myth of 'Safe Sex'." *Readers Digest*, August 1991.

– – –. "There Is No Safe Sex." *Newsweek*, 1 April 1991.

Painter, Kim. "Sex Habits of Young Women Change Little." *USA Today*, March 1991.

Pence, David M., M.D. *AIDS: A War We Can Win*, from The Grand Rapids Address. Forest Lake, Minn.: The Committee to Stop AIDS, 1988. Subsequently published in *Vital Speeches*, 1 February 1988.

Personal letter describing Planned Parenthood's Family Life Education Curriculum, K-12 (February 10, 1986), name confidential.

Pesman, Curtis. "Love and Sex in the 90s: Our National Survey." *Seventeen*, November 1991.

Planned Parenthood Federation of America, Inc., Education Department. *Emphasis* (Summer 1986) Issue title: "Consensus and Controversy: The Politics of Sexuality Education."

Emphasis (Autumn 1987) Issue title: "Religion and Sexuality: Current Perspectives."

– – –. *Is It o.k. for PPFA to say "No Way"?* New York: Department of Education, Planned Parenthood Federation of America, Inc., n.d.

"Predicting a News AIDS Toll." *U.S. News & World Report*, 13 May 1991.

Raeburn, Paul. "Virus May Be Linked to Genital Cancer." *Los Angeles Times*, 8 October 1983.

Rolfs, Robert T. and Nakashima, Ellyn K. "Epidemiology of Primary and Secondary Syphilis in the United States 1981–1989." *Journal of the American Medical Association*, 19 September 1991: 1432.

Ross, Walter S. "Our Unrecognized New VD Epidemic." *Readers Digest*, November 1979.

San Diego Union, 7 October 1991.

Scales, Peter, Ph.D. *Sexuality Education: The Value of Values*. New York: Emphasis Subscriber Service/Planned Parenthood Federation of America, Inc., 1983.

Sexuality Education: Definition and Discussion. New York: Department of Education, Planned Parenthood Federation of America, 1982.

Statistical Sources & Resources. A Publication of the Education Department LINK (Library and Information Network). New York: Planned Parenthood Federation of America, Inc., 1991.

The Value of Education in a Total Family Planning Program. New York: Department of Education, Planned Parenthood Federation of America, Inc., 1982.

Steinbrook, Robert. "AIDS Costs Will Nearly Double by 1994." *Los Angeles Times*, 20 June 1991.

Ting, Bauer, et al. "Nearly Half of Sexually Active College Women May Be HPV–Infected." *Medical Aspects of Human Sexuality*, March 1991: 49.

U.S. News & World Report, 2 June 1986.

Wallis, Claudia. "Viruses: Keys to Life and Death." *Time*, 3 November 1986.

Zenilman, Jonathan. "Sexually Transmitted Disease in Homosexual Adolescents." *Journal of Adolescent Health Care* 9, no. 2 (1988).

Index

Addendum

Does HIV infection equal the disease AIDS? According to the technical definitions, no. Unfortunately, the AIDS virus has been scientifically or medically politicized by certain interest groups, which has resulted in an inaccurate distinction between being HIV infected and having AIDS.

Usually, for a disease caused by bacteria or virus, once a person is infected, they have that disease. It is infection that equals having the disease; it is not having the end stages of that infection that equals having the disease. Thus, once a person is infected with the bacteria that causes Lyme disease they are diagnosed as *having* the disease identified by the presence of the bacteria.

The indispensable condition, or *sine qua non*, of AIDS is HIV infection. More precisely, AIDS is the external manifestation of an internal HIV infection. Thus in one sense it is inaccurate to imply that people who are "only HIV infected" do not have the disease of AIDS. In fact, they only lack the external manifestations or symptoms.

Nor does the fact that a vaccine may be developed for a specific disease mean that a person does not have the disease. To imply that people somehow do not have the disease of AIDS merely because they are only HIV infected and there may be a cure in the future is inaccurate.

Nor does the fact that a person is asymptomatic mean that they do not have a deadly disease called AIDS. There are many viral or bacterial-based diseases that, for a period of time, are asymptomatic and yet we say that the individual so infected has this or that disease. We do not say they are only infected with the specific virus causing the disease. For example, we never say that a person is Borrelia burgdorferi-infected; we simply say they have Lyme disease. It makes no difference whether a person is asymptomatic for a period of time or whether or not there will be a cure; they have Lyme disease from the point of infection.

In a similar manner, people *have* the disease of AIDS from the point of HIV infection, whether or not they are asymptomatic, whether or not they are in the end stages with external manifestations, or whether or not there will be a cure. For better or worse, "AIDS" is the common term for the disease; it is important that we do not make HIV infection any less a threat than it really is.

The Anker Series Booklets

(Eugene, Oreg.: Harvest House)

Other Books by Dr. John Ankerberg and Dr. John Weldon

Thieves of Innocence: A Parent's Handbook for Identifying New Age Religious Beliefs, Psychotherapeutic Techniques and Occult Practices in Public School Curriculums (Eugene, Oreg.: Harvest House).

Everything You Ever Wanted to Know About Mormonism (Eugene, Oreg.: Harvest House).

Cultwatch: What You Need to Know About Spiritual Deception, (Eugene, Oreg.: Harvest House).

Can You Trust Your Doctor? The Complete Guide to New Age Medicine and Its Threat to Your Family (Brentwood, Tenn.: Wolgemuth & Hyatt).

Rock Music's Powerful Messages (Chattanooga, Tenn.: Ankerberg Theological Research Institute).

One World: Bible Prophecy and the New World Order (Chicago: Moody).

The Secret Teachings of the Masonic Lodge: A Christian Perspective (Chicago: Moody).

When Does Life Begin? And 39 Other Tough Questions About Abortion (Brentwood, Tenn.: Wolgemuth & Hyatt).

Astrology: Do the Heavens Rule Our Destiny? (Eugene, Oreg.: Harvest House).

The Case for Jesus the Messiah: Incredible Prophecies That Prove God Exists (Eugene, Oreg.: Harvest House).

Christianity and the Secret Teachings of the Masonic Lodge (Chattanooga, Tenn.: Ankerberg Theological Research Institute).

Do the Resurrection Accounts Conflict? and What Proof Is There That Jesus Rose from the Dead? (Chattanooga, Tenn.: Ankerberg Theological Research Institute).